The Palgrave Lacan Series

Series Editors
Calum Neill, Edinburgh Napier University, Edinburgh, UK
Derek Hook, Duquesne University, Pittsburgh, USA

Jacques Lacan is one of the most important and influential thinkers of the 20th century. The reach of this influence continues to grow as we settle into the 21st century, the resonance of Lacan's thought arguably only beginning now to be properly felt, both in terms of its application to clinical matters and in its application to a range of human activities and interests. The Palgrave Lacan Series is a book series for the best new writing in the Lacanian field, giving voice to the leading writers of a new generation of Lacanian thought. The series will comprise original monographs and thematic, multi-authored collections. The books in the series will explore aspects of Lacan's theory from new perspectives and with original insights. There will be books focused on particular areas of or issues in clinical work. There will be books focused on applying Lacanian theory to areas and issues beyond the clinic, to matters of society, politics, the arts and culture. Each book, whatever its particular concern, will work to expand our understanding of Lacan's theory and its value in the 21st century.

Timothy Richardson

Nostalgia, Fantasy, and the Futures of Masculinity

palgrave
macmillan

Timothy Richardson
Department of English
The University of Texas at Arlington
Arlington, TX, USA

ISSN 2946-4196 ISSN 2946-420X (electronic)
The Palgrave Lacan Series
ISBN 978-3-032-23920-4 ISBN 978-3-032-23921-1 (eBook)
https://doi.org/10.1007/978-3-032-23921-1

Cover credit: CSA Images/Getty

This Palgrave Macmillan imprint is published by the registered company Springer Nature Switzerland AG
The registered company address is: Gewerbestrasse 11, 6330 Cham, Switzerland

For Sean Landry

Acknowledgments I need to begin by thanking my family for their support. They have lived through the kinds of grouchiness only a book can make. Huge thanks, too, to Ron Brooks and Nathan Gale, who suffered my texts and calls and video chats over most of the ideas in this book, who let me present with them at conferences, and whose encouragement saturates every page. And a special thank you to Kathryn Warren, whose responses and questions to early versions of two chapters pushed me to keep going, even though I wasn't sure.

Much of this book was prototyped through talks, presentations, etc., and wouldn't have been possible without the Lacan-centered LACK conference. I can't stress enough how valuable those meetings were and are. Additionally, I'm indebted to every scholar I've read (especially those cited directly, but also those who quietly sit constantly with me). Of course, some of what's here has grown out of earlier attempts at thinking through related questions, so I would also like to thank the following for allowing me to revisit earlier efforts in order to trouble, expand, and nuance: *Enculturation* for essay "The Authenticity of What's Next" and the audio essay "What Will Have Been Cool: Notes on Hauntological and Hypnogogic Music," *Hyperrhiz* for the text of part of the very short audio experiment "Ian Curtis," and *Popular Culture Review* for "The Looks of Men: Doubling and Nostalgia in Mad Men." Additionally, scattered in a couple of chapters of this book are ideas and some writing that appeared in a chapter titled "Home Bodies: Prosthetic People and Economies of Desire" in *Lacanian Perspectives on Blade Runner 2049*, published by this press.

In the end credits of many Universal Pictures horror classics are the words "A Good Cast is Worth Repeating." I thank my family again—Harper, Ben, and Laura—who are my causes. Their reservoirs of love and patience make anything I try to do feel possible.

Competing Interests The author has no competing interests to declare that are relevant to the content of this manuscript.

Contents

List of Figures

1
Introduction

A friend of mine is a seventh generation Texan who immigrated to New York City in the 1990s. Food-wise, this move marked a significant challenge. The Tex-Mex and other cuisines she had grown up with were no longer readily available in restaurants, so had to be cooked at home with ingredients sourced in complicated ways. Additionally, the kitchen space she had been accustomed to wasn't possible in a small apartment in a crowded city. So, she set herself the task of recreating the regional dishes of her childhood with what was available, in the space she had, with the cooking technologies that could physically fit there. This culinary translation exercise later yielded a successful blog and a series of cookbooks, all under the title of The Homesick Texan.

In her introduction to *The Homesick Texan Cookbook*, Lisa Fain (2011) states:

> Growing up, I didn't consider Texan food special, however, as it was simply what we ate. I guess you could say I took it for granted. So I was shocked when I moved to New York City and discovered that these beloved foods weren't readily available. Only then did I understand how unique and wonderful my home state's cuisine was. (p. 2)

T. Richardson, *Nostalgia, Fantasy, and the Futures of Masculinity*, The Palgrave Lacan Series, https://doi.org/10.1007/978-3-032-23921-1_1

With distance came a realization, and it's not a stretch to imagine that this *uniqueness* is *caused* by distance. Making authentic Texas food in Texas isn't much of a trick. Authenticity only matters once a copy is introduced against which an original may be compared. The cuisines of Texas can only become unique and wonderful once they're unavailable, so any cooking performance in the new place can be delicious and, since both she and the food aren't back there in Texas, in a weird way also a failure she can enjoy.

A couple of paragraphs later, Fain writes that "Not having easy access to Texan food made me feel homesick. But taking to my tiny New York City kitchen and cooking the foods that I had grown up with went far to help cure what ailed me" (p. 2). I like this last phrasing, *it went far to help*, as it stresses the distance (far) and that it only helps. Practice, performance, and participation maybe don't actually cure because that's not the point. Being here now, we enjoy the failure of trying to be there then. That's why we keep cooking.

Participation doesn't cure nostalgia as much as performs it. Contrasting with a kind of atrophied nostalgia that depends on collective symbols and slogans, Svetlana Boym (2002) suggests this other nostalgia "is more oriented toward an individual narrative that savors details and memorial signs, perpetually deferring homecoming itself" (p. 83). So, when The Homesick Texan recreates dishes from home with (often) different ingredients in a strange kitchen in a foreign state, she at once conjures the memory of home and performs its absence. And she tells stories about the origins of the featured dish and maybe also about the hunt for substitute ingredients, amplifying the distance through this summoning of particulars.

That distance is inherent to the activity and is especially obvious when the recipes are followed *in Texas*. I've had the honor of being a tester for a few dishes, performing the expatriate rituals from the home to which they point. But my West Texas is not her South Texas. And I've visited almost none of the places in Texas she catalogs as inspirational. To say "authentic Tex-Mex" or "authentic Texas barbeque" only makes sense outside of Texas, where the nostalgic detail is approximate and every attempt is at once a failure and, hopefully, close enough to enjoy. In Texas, we'd have to get regional, local, familial, dicing more and more finely. These are the stories of origins that introduce the cookbooks' recipes. The necessity of distance, of difference, is also what has allowed The Homesick Texan to move back to Texas and remain homesick.

Early in *The Future of Nostalgia*, Boym (2002) reminds us that the word nostalgia was coined by Swiss doctor Johannes Hofer in his 1688 dissertation for the medical condition triggered by a longing for one's homeland. Literally, it's a sickness caused by being separated from home (p. 24). In these early medical studies Boym describes, "Gastronomic and auditory nostalgia were of particular importance. Swiss scientists found that rustic mothers' soups, thick village milk and the folk melodies of Alpine valleys were particularly conducive to triggering a nostalgic reaction in Swiss soldiers" (p. 25). The gastronomic addresses all the senses, so the pull can be especially strong. Smells and flavors are what I think of first, but the look of a hard taco (for instance), the crunch at biting, and the texture of the food in my mouth may evoke both a geographic and temporal distance. Even if I return home, what I find there often reminds me of what used to be there, when I was younger and, maybe only in my recollection, happier.

Dr. Hofer didn't just talk about food inducing homesickness, but sound, too. For those of us who haven't been to war (and for many who have), nostalgia points back most often to a time when life was simpler, and music is very portable. The "folk melodies of Alpine valleys" have become, for us, collaged retro sounds in music, the staging of vintage stereo systems, surging production of new vinyl records, and the cobbling of personal playlists like old mixtapes in an effort to return to a temporal home as much as a geographical one, or at least to pretend. Each insists on embodied experiences as a performance of some distance right now.

The entertainment industries have taken note. For food, cooking shows (competitive and not) have long been evergreen programming on television, and I often find myself selecting a free, ad-supported channel on the smart tv to watch decades-old pan-frying. Beyond the gastronomic, old music, movies, and television programs are now immediately available for streaming. At the same time, screens of all sizes are filled with new remakes of older films, prequels and sequels to beloved franchises, and cinematic universes devoted to the stories I grew up with. The marketability of the repackaged past means that product and media creators constantly look for warm feelings to exploit in retro products—shrunken video arcade machines for the home, audio cassettes, adult happy meals—while algorithms collate new and remastered old songs together onto the same safe, familiar playlist.

Marketing has always been about persuasion, but it has never been so insistently temporal. *Nostalgia, Fantasy, and the Futures of Masculinity* investigates relationships between nostalgia, fantasy, capital, and masculinity, with special emphasis placed on how these relations are deployed when we talk (and argue) about the future.

Time, Time, Time[1]

The introduction to a special issue of *Rhetoric Society Quarterly* declares that "time is foundational to the design of rhetorical theory and practice" (Bjork & Buhre, 2021, p. 178). As far back as the fourth century BCE, Aristotle assigned three temporalities to rhetoric: the forensic past, the epideictic present, and the deliberative future. But regardless of the time to which it is directed, rhetoric concentrates on what potential to persuade exists *right now* (Aristotle calls this potential *dunamis*) as we assign guilt in the courtroom, praise a person in a speech, or pass legislation for a desired future. This concentration on the present is also the basis of psychoanalytic intercession. While my academic background is broadly in rhetoric studies, the theoretical apparatuses for this book are primarily psychoanalytic, as they offer unique methods for exposing fissures—the gaps I'll argue that make space for potential—and for exploiting these to create occasions for change. Psychoanalysis is directed toward intervening *now* to relieve suffering. And we are suffering.

Though my approach is principally psychoanalytic, the voices informing the work of this book are many and insistent. Svetlana Boym's now-classic *The Future of Nostalgia* is a touchstone. Her elaborations on the kinds and consequences of nostalgia are particularly important, as are

---

[1] Here, I'm referencing the excellent Bangles 1987 cover of the Simon and Garfunkel 1966 song "A Hazy Shade of Winter."

her warnings. The collisions she describes between nostalgia and technology lead to the messiness of capitalized nostalgia that much of this book works to highlight.

Throughout this work, I use phrases like "capitalism" and "neoliberal capitalism." By these I primarily mean what Steven Shaviro (2015) lays out in *No Speed Limit: Three Essays on Accelerationism*. Beginning the list with (1) the transfer of wealth from most of us to the richest people and (2) privatizing as much of the commons as possible, he finishes up with:

3. The extraction…of a surplus from all social activities: not only from production (as in the classical Marxist model of capitalism) but from circulation and consumption as well. Capital accumulation proceeds not only by direct exploitation but also by rent-seeking, by debt collection, and by outright expropriation ("primitive accumulation").
4. The subjection of all aspects of life to the so-called discipline of the market. This is equivalent, in more traditional Marxist terms, to the "real subsumption" by capital of all aspects of life: leisure as well as labor. Even our sleep is now organized in accordance with the imperatives of production and capital accumulation.
5. The redefinition of human beings as private owners of their own "human capital." Each person is thereby, as Michel Foucault puts it, forced to become "an entrepreneur of himself." In such circumstances, we are continually obliged to market ourselves, to "brand" ourselves, to maximize the return on our "investment" (p. 7–8).

Of particular interest are these last three: the merging of the private and public, wealth extraction from leisure, human capital, and so on. While I'm compelled by arguments that we're moving (or perhaps have even already moved) from a capitalist economy to a new kind of technocracy (a techno-or-neofeudalism that equates capital with efficiency and measures success by excess[2]), as of now, at least, this possible shifting only amplifies the individual consumer's feeling of buying into a system

[2] Neofeudalism is partly a refinement of modes in which, as in Shaviro above, "Capital accumulation proceeds not only by direct exploitation but also by rent-seeking, by debt collection, and by outright expropriation" through governmental exploits as well as theft. See, for instance, Varoufakis (2024) and Dean (2025).

that particularizes and isolates the subject as much as it disperses the person into a demographic. The use of *capitalism* throughout this book is thus primarily consumer-focused, as capitalism itself possibly becomes a fantasy covering a darker situation.

Likewise, Mark Fisher's insights on capitalism, music, and their intersection are an essential basis for my own thoughts on music and other media, along with their relation to the discourse of capitalism. *Capitalist Realism* (2008/2022), as he calls it, is pervasive.[3] Additionally, his assertion (2013/2022) in *Ghosts of My Life* that "there's an increasing sense that culture has lost the ability to grasp and articulate the present. Or it could be that, in one very important sense, there is no present to grasp and articulate any more," is extended to discussions of the future (p. 9).

In calling capitalism a discourse, I follow Jacques Lacan's addition to his four primary discourses—master, university, hysteric, analyst—with a commanding fifth capitalist kind that may replace the master for us. Oscillating between the specific and structural, the Lacanian flavor of psychoanalytic thought demonstrates that what is often assumed to be personal is not only overly determined by what is usually called culture, but that hegemonic structures are sustained by a kind of private enjoyment. Essential to my elaborations of nostalgic symptoms are insights offered by Mari Ruti, Alenka Zupančič, and Slavoj Žižek, among many others.

In displays of deliberative rhetoric, two recent American presidents have sloganeered a nostalgia-inflected future to either a call to a particular constituency ("Make America Great Again") or to promote expensive, long-term government investment in national infrastructure ("Build Back Better"). Both look back to near mythic times in American history (the Gilded Age of the late nineteenth Century and the golden baby-boom years of the 1950s, or the New Deal of the 1930s) as models for action in the present in order to mold a desired future. That mythic quality is fostered by distance and memory. But in a world of immediate digital recall and same-day delivery, there may no longer be any distance.

[3] Less cited, but no less affecting for my project, are the personal discussions across his work, as well as his death. While I didn't know him, we had a few mutual friends, were around the same age, and his loss—along with a close friend of mine whom we lost at around the same time and to whom this book is dedicated—haunts these pages.

Some questions that *Nostalgia, Fantasy, and the Futures of Masculinity* takes up are: What happens when pasts, via technologies and media productions tailored to capture our memories and capitalize on our youths, are rendered almost wholly present? In what ways can the subsequent reinforcement of outdated values and toxic commonplaces be resisted? What can we say now about the future that isn't just some version of futures we used to imagine? What can we do now to escape a vast present caught up in the oscillation of capitalism.

The Systemic is Personal

To address these and other questions, this book explores music, television shows, films, and other media products that somehow reinscribe the problems of the past and often project them into the future, but that may also work to short-circuit that process. One of these problems is masculinity, and an ongoing concern of this book is the ways in which both nostalgia and its capitalistic exploitation resemble and promote masculine structures in both the popular notion of manhood and in a specific Lacanian psychoanalytic dispensation.

There is—apparently—a crisis in masculinity. In her *Washington Post* opinion essay "Men are lost. Here's a map out of the wilderness," Christine Emba maps some of the more recent challenges to knowing how to be a man: the rise of unemployment among young men, as jobs shift away from manufacturing and toward soft skills requiting a college degree; the rise in dating standards among women, as women become less dependent on marriage for security and children; etc. And there is a concomitant rise in "deaths of despair" (almost 3 out of every 4) from substance abuse or suicide (2023). While for the older men there's old-school gold to be bought, one response of the market is the insinuation of new kinds of money (cryptocurrencies) to make up for a lack of the traditional stuff, giving rise to the crypto bro (Cassino, 2023, 2024). And then deposed Fox News darling Tucker Carlson touts the unobvious benefits of sunning your testicles to increase testosterone with the "purchase [of] in-home devices such as light beds, lamps, lasers, and infrared saunas, which range in price from hundreds to thousands of dollars" (Karlis, 2022).[4]

These are a few of the symptoms of today's crisis, but Emba admits it's not a new problem, pointing to American concerns from as early as 1835 and into the early 1900s. As culture shifts and expectations change, following the real-man script is challenging. We should likely read complaints about "woke-ness" and DEI in our popular media and politics as anxiety regarding these shifts. As Calum Neill (2020) rightly claims, "It has always been difficult to be a man, insofar as the ideal of masculinity is precisely that: an ideal" (p. 11). But the ideal used to change more slowly. Now, with so much available—in movies, on television, in social media—and so much contradiction, the crisis is in crisis.

What Jacques Lacan delineates as the masculine subject (via what he calls sexuation) is a kind of failure that depends on fantasy structures to maintain a stumbling functioning. The structure of fantasy closely resembles the structures of media and other products, which is why the fantastic idea can be sold back to me. And if that fantasy is nostalgia for times "when men were men" (a time that, in fact, never existed), then there is already a demand for these products.

In the preface to his 1993 book chronicling the history and pleasures of cigarette smoking, *Cigarettes are Sublime*, Richard Klein (1995) begins:

> My motives for writing this book are complex. They certainly had their origin in my urgent desire to stop smoking. In order not to do it any more, I felt I needed above all to understand the specific nature and determine the general conditions of my habit. That need, in turn, led me to the question that shaped this book's conception: What prompts nearly a billion people in the world, every day, to light up and inhale, when they know it is bad for their health? (p. IX)

[4] Amanda Marcotte (2025), in the pointedly-titled "Don't blame women for men's loneliness. Blame capitalism" for *Salon*, claims "it's time to look at how male loneliness has been monetized by all manner of seedy actors who have every incentive to discourage men from making changes to improve their lives. Men's ability to adapt to modernity is being stymied by propagandists and grifters, who persuade men to adopt anti-social behavior, because doing so is incredibly profitable" (paragraph 9).

Regarding nostalgia and its marketing, my feelings are much the same. First, it often feels bad.[5] What began as annoyance at hearing music by The Cure piped into a nearby chain grocery store (The Cure have never made grocery store music) has become frustration at streaming algorithms feeding me music and movies I've already heard or seen (or, worse, *feel* like I've heard and seen), constant television-show reboots, endless cinematic universes, et cetera. And the methods through which culture is piped to me are almost frictionless. The technologies of consuming are no longer demanding and confusing in the way that programming a video-cassette recorder was for my dad, as the move to the cloud—along with the introduction of algorithms and artificial intelligence—takes that labor offsite and makes it invisible. In more and more instances, I just have to say out loud what I want. The future of "friction-free capitalism" that Bill Gates (1995) foresaw in the 1990s is here (p. 183). And it's boring.

I say *frustration*, but I also can't help but gorge myself on the comfort food of this easy nostalgia buffet. Hearing "Love Cats" in the International aisle at the grocery store is inviting, comfortable, and I find myself singing along while considering salsas. Of course, this isn't a new phenomenon. I remember rolling my eyes back in our previous century when hearing an Eagles song at the grocery store, so I have to allow for the possibility that part of the frustration could be recognizing myself as one of the old folks to whom grocery-store music is set to appeal. But as music, films, and television programs began to depend on properties from my youth to such an extent that living in the past feels like the only possible present, it's difficult not to feel stuck. Production designer David Warren's offhand comment about his work on Terry Gilliam's *The Zero Theorem* (2014), that it offers a "bubblegum dystopia," feels more generally applicable (Stubbs, 2023).[6] There is no nutritional value to bubblegum, but I keep chewing.

---

[5] I've seen Echo and the Bunnymen perform maybe a dozen times over the past few decades and, while they still sound strong, I can't help but feel that my money and time have been spent reliving instead of living and that at best what I've gained is a new t-shirt. And this is true beyond my personal choices.

[6] The film *Barbie* (2023), for all of its laudable gender politics and outlandish excitement, offers a bubblegum dystopia (Mould, 2024) (Nguyen, 2024).

What follows is (in part) an attempt "to understand the specific nature and determine the general conditions of my habit." For this reason, while much of my project works through structural impasses pertaining to nostalgia, fantasy, capitalism, and masculinity, I am implicated throughout. The rampant use of personal pronouns in this project is (in part) a way to recognize that my view is only partial and that I'm always already culpable. This has made the book sometimes uncomfortable to write, both because it can appear self-indulgent and, possibly, because it is self-indulgent. But, glossing both Pierre Bourdieu and Donna Haraway, Johnathan Sterne (2012) maintains that "knowers must place themselves in relation to what it is they want to know: they must account for their own positions and prejudices, lest scholars misattribute them as qualities of the object of study"(p. 4). Decentering the (this) cisgendered white male perspective is an ongoing challenge, and consistently drawing attention to my own investment and guilt insists on my partiality.[7]

According to Kenneth Burke (1945/1969), the representative anecdote "contains *in nuce* the terminological structure that is evolved in conformity with it.... Thus the anecdote is in a sense a *summation*, containing implicitly what the system that is developed from it contains explicitly" (p. 60). As representational anecdotes both precede and summarize the explicit content of the work, my use of the personal alongside other, popular examples (hopefully) shapes the discussion in ways that are always obviously contingent and partial. Following Alenka Zupančič (2017), the goal "is thus not neutrality, but the capacity of theory to occupy a singular, specific point of view within the situation. In this sense, the objectivity is linked here to the very capacity of being 'partial' or 'partisan'" (p. 4). That is, this book represents my thinking through some problems that are as personal as they are structural, so it would be a mistake to assume a privileged, "objective" narrative place above these issues. I am a middle-aged cis-gendered white guy talking

[7] When using his own dreams as examples for analysis, Sigmund Freud famously stopped short of real embarrassment or disclosures that were too personal, explaining "I could draw closer together the threads in the material revealed by the analysis, and I could then show that they converge upon a single nodal point, but considerations of a personal and not of a scientific nature prevent my doing so in public" (Freud, 1980, p. 15). I plead the same.

(in part) about problems with (which are also problems of) middle-aged cis-gendered white guys.

In *How to Make Art at the End of the World*, Natalie Loveless (2019) writes: "To take anecdote as a storytelling practice seriously, as a way of acknowledging the webs of indebtedness that are constitutive of and give rise to any academic life, is first to anchor one's theory within the unpredictable affective terrain of daily life" (66). To bring the anecdotal into larger social discussions is also to assert, with Jeff Rice (2021), that

> The personal, too, is a force within networks producing meaning and one that deserves details. In any given moment—whether it is textual, political, emotional, economical, educational—there is the person writing about the moment and the person experiencing the moment. That person interacts with the subject matter, as well. The individual, as reader, writer, parent, beer drinker, foodie, traveler, academic, and so forth, is also an actor in a given network of interactions. (p. 8)

The personal is a force within networks.[8] There are individual and systemic stakes in my (and our) understanding and resisting of nostalgic appeals and capitalist exploitations that both shape and are shaped by a masculinity specified through failure. Demonstrating this is the job of the book that follows.

What Will Have Been

Nothing sparks nostalgic feelings like hearing a song I loved in high school. Listening to Cocteau Twins now also means listening to them through a down-market personal cassette player on late-night post-football-game band trips, returning home after another loss. Drawing from Mark Fisher and many others, the first chapter considers popular

---

[8] Žižek (1992) makes the negative version of this point when he asserts:

> the very social law that, as a kind of neutral set of rules, should limit our aesthetic self-creation and deprive us of a part of our enjoyment on behalf of solidarity, is always already penetrated by an obscene, "pathological," surplus enjoyment. The point is thus not that the split public/private is not possible, but that it is possible only on condition that the very domain of the public law is "smeared" by an obscene dimension of "private" enjoyment.... (p. 159).

music and the nostalgia it can elicit by thinking through some repercussions of the music streaming archive—Spotify, etc.—as all music becomes *contemporary* music algorithmically gathered onto a common infinite playlist. At the same time, technologies of the past—cassette tapes, hi-fi stereos, etc.—have become fetishized as (often digitally) reproducible *pasts* that provoke nostalgic reactions even in audiences who weren't alive during the times evoked. This apparently tame kind of nostalgia (here performed through anecdote as well as a theoretical investigation) points toward how fantasy becomes a mechanism for political and economic exploitation, as discussed via Lacan and others in the next chapter.

Mass media is in the fantasy business. The third chapter follows fantasy to other circumstances by examining the functions of genre in its production and maintenance. Beginning with classic *Star Trek*, genre fantasy media, and fan culture and ending by defining the psychoanalytic fantasy structure that late capitalism exploits, the chapter works through collecting, cosplay, and film and television genres to demonstrate how they simultaneously teach and police stasis. Drawing heavily from the work of Donna Haraway, Ursula K. Le Guin, Todd McGowan, Steven Shaviro, Colette Soler, Stijn Vanheule, and Alenka Zupančič, it then connects this stasis to the mechanisms whereby "personal" fantasy (understood through a psychoanalytic lens) becomes accessible to marketing strategies and exploitable worldviews (and the business of fantasy beyond media). Capitalist discourse mines the past and exploits the present by making promises about an infinitely deferred future. Fantasy is its engine.

The fourth chapter considers the function of women forced to operate as tools for the servicing of both late capitalism and masculine fantasy via three case studies. Through the development that Jacques Lacan called *sexuation* and elaborations by Isabel Millar, Mari Ruti, Slavoj Žižek, and others, this chapter looks closely at a recent past performed by the tv series *Mad Men* (2007) and two recent futures proffered by the films *Her* and *Ex Machina* to discern how circulations of late capitalism map to masculine fantasy and how static, nostalgic ideas of the feminine promote both.

Continuing this discussion, the fifth chapter details how women may function as props for supporting masculine fantasy, especially (as Sarah Sharma argues) the fantasy of escaping into a better future. The dystopic science fiction of the two *Blade Runner* films (1982, 2017) and the post-apocalypse of *Mad Max: Fury Road* (2015) demonstrate that masculine fantasy is a set of conventions very similar to genre conventions, as a received script is reinforced with every iteration. But iteration (perhaps) makes intercession possible. The fantasy of escape—from conflict, from environment, etc.—is intimately tied to the fantastic support on which capital depends (e.g. real-life billionaires and their rockets).

One recurring concern of fantasy is *authenticity*. Is this authentic music? Are our costumes authentic? Can we make authentic (robotic, digital) fake people? Where the preceding chapters point toward the importance of authenticity regarding food, music, genre fantasy, fan culture, set staging, and gender roles, the sixth chapter argues that pleas for authenticity are very often nostalgic calls for comfort (or for the exotic in comfortable surroundings). Roving from strip-mall Mexican fare to comic books to sex dolls and handmade infants, the chapter looks for the failures of authenticity as possible sites of exploitation, as opportunities to toss a stick into the spokes of the accelerating cycles of capitalist discourse.

Disrupting the stasis of the infinite present that is bolstered by nostalgia and the accelerated circulation of late capitalism is the goal. But that's hard. Returning to complications of Mark Fisher's capitalist realism, the concluding chapter looks to ways to intercede in the cycles, to break the static long present and allow for the possibility of (at least) thinking about the future differently. Once again, Mari Ruti is crucial for the connection of capital and enjoyment, but so are practical investments like Shannon Mattern's work on understanding (and using) established infrastructure like public libraries differently, Keller Easterling's design work that foregrounds medium (not product), and especially Natalie Loveless's promotion of research-creation as a valuable activity for engaging with new knowledge. These folks (and others) offer methods for interceding in the frantic flow that maintains the experience of stasis and develop strategies for generating new possible futures. I also offer some tentative, local, provisional suggestions for how to (maybe) effect change. But, as Mattern and Easterling and Loveless demonstrate (but rarely say), the point is pretty much to give up on the personal, the individual, the essential core of the self that is a fundamental fantasy. This is the fantasy that capitalism, masculinity, and nostalgia exploit equally, and often all at once. The goal instead is to dedicate myself (at least) to *working*, to *helping*, to *doing* without allegiance to a final, marketable, useful product. Of course, having tenure at a large university lets me do that. At least for now.

References

Bjork, C., & Buhre, F. (2021). Resisting temporal regimes, imagining just temporalities. *Rhetoric Society Quarterly, 51*(3), 177–181.

Boym, S. (2002). *The future of nostalgia*. Basic Books.

Burke, K. (1969). *A grammar of motives*. University of California Press.

Cassino, D. (2023). Crypto, meme stocks, and threatened masculinity. *Contexts, 22*(2), 18–23.

Cassino, D. (2024, September 20). Opinion: Why crypto bros love Trump. *Washington Post*. https://www.washingtonpost.com/opinions/2024/09/20/trump-cryptocurrency-poll-masculinity/

Dean, J. (2025). *Capital's grave: Neofeudalism and the new class struggle*. Verso Books.

Emba, C. (2023, July 10). Opinion: Men are lost. Here's a map out of the wilderness. *Washington Post*. https://www.washingtonpost.com/opinions/2023/07/10/christine-emba-masculinity-new-model/

Fain, L. (2011). *The homesick Texan cookbook*. Hachette Books.

Fisher, M. (2022). *Ghosts of my life: Writings on depression, Hauntology and lost futures* (2nd ed.). Zero Books.

Freud, S. (1980). *On dreams*. Norton.

Gates, B. (1995). *The road ahead* (with Illustrated ed.). Viking Press.

Karlis, N. (2022, April 21). Tucker Carlson hawks "testicle tanning" to boost testosterone. Experts say it may do the opposite. *Salon*. https://www.salon.com/2022/04/21/tucker-carlson-testicle-tanning/

Klein, R. (1995). *Cigarettes are sublime*. Duke University Press Books.

Loveless, N. (2019). *How to make art at the end of the world: A manifesto for research-creation*. Duke University Press Books.

Marcotte, A. (2025, November 17). *Don't blame women for men's loneliness. Blame capitalism.* Salon.Com. https://www.salon.com/2025/11/17/dont-blame-women-for-mens-loneliness-blame-capitalism/?utm_source=website&utm_medium=social&utm_campaign=ogshare&utm_content=og

Mould, O. (2024, August 2). Bubblegum Dystopia: The Sweet Decay of Late-Stage Capitalism. *taCity*. https://tacity.co.uk/2024/08/02/bubblegum-dystopia-the-sweet-decay-of-late-stage-capitalism/

Neill, C. (2020). Masculinity in crisis: Myth, fantasy and the promise of the raw. *Psychoanalysis, Culture & Society, 25*(1), 4–17.

Nguyen, S. (2024, August 10). "Bubblegum dystopia": What it is and how it's creeping into pop culture—And reality. *The Daily Dot*. https://www.dailydot.com/pop-culture/bubblegum-dystopia/

Rice, J. (2021). *Authentic writing*. University of Pittsburgh Press.

Shaviro, S. (2015). *No speed limit: Three essays on accelerationism.* University of Minnesota Press.

Sterne, J. (Ed.). (2012). *The sound studies reader*. Routledge.

Stubbs, P. (2023, February 25). *Bubblegum Dystopia.* Dreams: The Terry Gilliam Fanzine. https://www.gilliamdreams.com/ziptdw2.htm

Varoufakis, Y. (2024). *Technofeudalism: What killed capitalism.* Melville House.

Žižek, S. (1992). *Looking awry: An introduction to Jacques Lacan through popular culture* (Reprint ed.). The MIT Press.

Žižek, S. (2007). How to read Lacan (1st edition). Norton & Company.

Zupančič, A. (2017). *What is sex?* The MIT Press.

2

The Old Sound of Now

> I exist on the best terms I can.
> The past is now part of my future,
> The present is well out of hand.
> —Joy Division, "Heart and Soul"

The evening I first heard Ian Curtis sing was also the evening I learned that he had been dead for four years.

"I've been waiting for a guide to come and take me by the hand" are the first lines of Joy Division's first album,1979's *Unknown Pleasures*. Hearing those lines and that news at pretty much the same time evoked the kind of negative capability that sensitive 15-year-olds are probably perfectly made for.

The opening for this chapter began as part of a very short experimental audio piece Richardson, T. (2021). Ian Curtis. *Hyperrhiz: New Media Cultures, 23*. https://doi.org/10.20415/hyp/023.r07. The end of this chapter is based on the text of my audio essay Richardson, T. (2022). What Will Have Been Cool: Notes on Hauntological and Hypnogogic Music. *Enculturation.net*. https://www.enculturation.net/what_will_have_been_cool.

T. Richardson, *Nostalgia, Fantasy, and the Futures of Masculinity*, The Palgrave Lacan Series, https://doi.org/10.1007/978-3-032-23921-1_2

I remember sitting at my friend Mike's house. He had just gotten the only two albums—copied to a blank cassette, one on each side—by the band that New Order used to be. Before digital ubiquity, cassettes were the best way we had to copy and disseminate music. The coincidence of a large air force base near our West Texas town meant an influx of kids from all over the country. They brought their music with them and were happy to share, as long as we sprung for blank Maxells.

My connection with Ian Curtis has always been through a mediation that drew attention to itself. There's the obvious distance that recording allows, so that someone who is dead can sing five years later. The tape hiss of copies of copies of cassettes made listening feel underground and vaguely elicit. The sound engineering of Martin Hannett meant that a live Joy Division was very different, which we found out years later as gig recordings surfaced and were eventually released. And Curtis did very few interviews and never talked about his process, so reading books by people who knew him—his wife and band mates—or by critics who listened closely was my only way in.

The band's first single, "Transmission," was a song I heard later, only after digesting those two albums. It sums up the dissonance of time and mediation this way: "Staying in the same place, just staying out the time/Touching from a distance, further all the time." I've never finished reading a book or watching a film about Ian Curtis, have always stopped well short of his death. Ian Curtis killed himself on May 18, 1980. He was 23 years old. At that age, he had a wife and a daughter and band that was just about to start an American tour. Years after first hearing him, I found out that he had suffered from epilepsy as well as depression and had often been in a great deal of pain. When I first heard him sing, though, I only knew that he had died. And that he was also here, right now.

It's likely that there is no time in our lives that music matters more than when we're teenagers. As we try to define our selves against whatever we've received up to that point, songs become personal and genres become teams. I'm now at an age where popular music from my teenage years is the music played at grocery stores to make me feel comfortable. I don't like that.

This chapter considers the mediation, performance, and marketing of nostalgia through music and identity, with an ear toward describing the temporal distance on which nostalgia sometimes relies and the mechanisms by which that distance is collapsed in order to render every instance of every song an occasion *right now*.

Recombinatorial Delirium

I have sometimes liked to ask students about what kinds of music were popular when. If we start well before they were born—with the end of the twentieth Century—and go back by decade, depending on their parents, the lists may run something like Grunge and Hip-Hop in the 1990s, maybe New Wave and Hair Metal in the 80s, possibly Punk or Disco in the 70s, maybe something about hippies before that, then something called Rock and Roll, and that's about as far as we get.

When I ask them about the first two decades of this century, though, they're usually quiet for a moment. After a while, someone might say "still Hip-Hop" and others will say something like Indie or Post Rock and maybe a few will complain that those aren't really things. Often, instead of genres, they'll turn to artists: Beyoncé, Radiohead, Taylor Swift, and so on. At some point, someone may suggest that we're still too close to it to name it. Maybe, but we knew what New Wave was in the 1980s and people labeled Grunge in the 1990s. It was on fashion runways.

Eventually, someone will say there wasn't a sound and someone else will say "It's everything!"

What if they are both right? Since the beginning of this century, much of all the popular music ever recorded has become easily and instantly accessible. The move to digital (and the remastering that sometimes entails) has allowed a flattening of scenes such that more or less every piece of music is exactly as available as any other. New and old tracks are jumbled to stream anywhere I am, often sacrificing any prior context in favor of their present playlist. It's as if the algorithm extends and possibly perfects what David Toop (1995) describes as the disco DJ's innovation in his 1995 book *Ocean of Sound*, when "Songs became liquid. They became vehicles for improvisation, or source materials, field recordings almost, that could be reconfigured or remixed to suit the future" (p. 43). We are living in the future. All music is now contemporary music.

One possible result is that, when everything suddenly becomes always available, it is more difficult for new work to find a critical mass and become a prevailing or dominant style. Niche music or older works that used to be difficult to find are suddenly as available as the broadest pop, and this work may sound fresh enough that anything very new could be lost in the flood of the new-to-me. As all of these get arranged on playlists and streamed—often by algorithms that have mined my data for educated guesses about my tastes and mood—the new context isn't one of influences and styles as much as it is my purchase history and likes on social media. The past becomes a tabulated, commercial enterprise and the present is its marketplace.

The prospect that the sound of the first decade of the 2000s was both everything and nothing dismays Mark Fisher who, in *Ghosts of My Life* (2014/2022), submits:

> Imagine any record released in the past couple of years being beamed back in time to, say, 1995 and played on the radio. It's hard to think that it will produce any jolt in the listeners. On the contrary, what would be likely to shock our 1995 audience would be the very recognisability of the sounds: would music really have changed so little in the next 17 years? Contrast this with the rapid turnover of styles between the 1960s and the 90s: play a jungle record from 1993 to someone in 1989 and it would have sounded like something so new that it would have challenged them to rethink what music was, or could be. While 20th-century experimental culture was seized by a recombinatorial delirium, which made it feel as if newness was infinitely available, the 21st century is oppressed by a crushing sense of finitude and exhaustion. It doesn't feel like the future. Or, alternatively, it doesn't feel as if the 21st century has started yet. (p. 7–8)

Fisher's assessment is pretty dour. This isn't the future we were promised. But to be fair, perhaps the twentieth Century set up unrealistic expectations for music in the twenty-first Century.

The potential of radical difference—or at least strikingly new combinations—that Fisher lauds is as much a consequence of the confluence of new technologies and new markets as it is individual genius. That experimental culture he is nostalgic for maps nicely to the invention of recording and playback devices. In 1930, Igor Stravinsky anticipates the creative flow of a DJ's turntablism (kind of) when he predicts that "It would be of the greatest interest to create music specifically for the phonograph, a music whose true image—its original sound—could only be preserved through mechanical reproduction. This would well be the ultimate goal for the phonographic composers of the future" (Taylor et al., 2012, p 113). And the global introduction of magnetic tape immediately following World War II sets the conditions for avant-garde and experimental musical genres such as musique concrète (wherein recorded sounds are processed and used as material for musical compositions), quite literally performing a "recombinatorial delirium." The same magnetic tape also allows multitracking, easy edits, higher fidelity (paving the way for the move from shellac to polyvinyl for records), consumer hi-fi setups, and home and portable recording equipment that lowers the barrier to entry for many.

Coincidentally, roughly the same decade that marks the wide adoption of magnetic tape sees, if not the invention of, then the recognition and naming of the teenager as a distinct group with their own affordances, first in the United States as heralded by the "Teen-Age Bill of Rights" in 1945 (Cohen, 1945), and then as an export to the rest of the world.[1]

Certainly, the very experimental music produced in the twentieth Century wasn't aimed at teens (John Cage's "Williams Mix" was not a hit among sixteen-year-olds), nor were they very likely to run across it. But these new teenagers were increasingly consuming music that would have been impossible before the technology that allowed its capture, manipulation, and distribution. The same recording technology used by the experimentalists to explore new possibilities in sound manipulation and trace the contours of what could be considered musical also allows people who are not musicians to nonetheless handle music, have music on demand, and makes music increasingly shareable, just in time for a constituency with leisure and at least enough cash to sometimes buy and

[1] See, for instance, the 2013 documentary *Teenage* for both video evidence and a fantastic musical score.

trade records, tapes, and compact disks. My point is that the decades Fisher points to are also decades in which product and customer were becoming so closely aligned that much of the marketing of recorded music was often also the marketing to and of the teenager.

We still have recorded music (and teenagers, of course), and the digital revolution of the late 1990s into the 2000s promised even more democratization of the means and ability to produce and consume. But, for Fisher, twenty-first Century popular music—and, by extension, popular culture as a whole—was and (probably) still is in a depressing kind of stasis in which the present consists of little but the recycled and commodified past. He worries that "the very distinction between past and present is breaking down" so that "cultural time has folded back on itself, and the impression of linear development has given way to a strange simultaneity" (2014).

The digital music archive is such a strange simultaneity. Practically every piece of music ever recorded is available *right now* for around a dollar each. Much of it can be streamed like a personalized radio station for a relatively low monthly buy-in. I don't purchase much music anymore; I subscribe to a Service.

This colossal archive—into which services like Spotify and Apple Music are portals—is only recently available, but its effects have been massive. With the virtual elimination of the need for physical media, there is no scarcity of product—outside of artificial limits on downloads or plays—and new work and old work are worth exactly the same and are found on the same algorithmically-produced playlists. In the presence of this bounty of music (and the wealth it produces for companies), how is the "new" even possible, given the variety of what is already here? Anything is new if it's new to you.

Of course, it isn't that the past shouldn't be (and isn't) valued. Working with, through, and against the past is essential for innovation. Fisher (2009) admits this elsewhere, echoing T.S. Eliot's famous argument about tradition: "The new defines itself in response to what is already established; at the same time, the established has to reconfigure itself in response to the new" (p. 3). We come to terms with our past best through its relationship to and rivalry with the present; this is how we recognize innovation. His complaint is, rather, that instead of being caught in a *recombinatorial delirium*, the flattened commercial past has become a placeholder for an evacuated present. We don't remix so much as collect.

Additionally, "Capitalism," Fisher argues, "subsumes and consumes all of previous history: [this is] one effect of its 'system of equivalence' which can assign all cultural objects, whether they are religious iconography, pornography, or *Das Kapital*, a monetary value" (p. 4). Once cultural value is translated to monetary value, any trading takes place on an equal field and any one object can be substituted for any other. A dollar per song is an example of this translation, insofar as it allows any song onto the playlist for the exact same buy-in by stripping it of any other context. This system of equivalences, the flattening of the past and its packaging for and as the present, replaces innovation with metonymic iteration.

This is how our new notion of "normal" is generated and maintained. Difference is subsumed by the market as another attribute among many, all priced to go. This new normal is predicated on immediacy, leading Anna Kornbluh (2024) to assert that "The twenty-first-century concentration on circulation, with its premium on flow, conditions immediacy as cultural style that immanentizes presence, eclipses relay, and negates mediation" such that "Speed is, of course, the preeminent colloquial connotation of 'immediacy,' and flatness is the dimension of smooth flow" (p. 30). The effect of the flattening of the past and present via the system of equivalences that late capitalism *is* is a kind of frantic circulation in a great simultaneity, a common place, wherein the past and present are commingled, and nothing is lost because everything can be counted.[2]

And we can subscribe to that accounting.

Perhaps ironically, the music industry helped push us toward not buying music, starting with the practically forced conversion from analog records and cassettes to compact discs. As writer (and drummer for the band Galaxie 500) Damon Krukowski (2017) recounts:

[2] In the psychoanalytic terms of the succeeding chapters, this new normal is a kind of psychosis made ordinary, where, according to Marie-Hélène Brousse (2013), "it is super social behaviour. It's an absolute submission…to common uses, to the commonplace, as defined by the median of the bell curve. Statistics are no longer envisaged in the framework of probability, but take on the value of certitude" (p. 27).

> Of course, the music industry loved CDs. No one could fold, mutilate, or lick the metallic discs sealed inside their plastic "jewel cases," eliminating the damaged paper sleeves and scratched vinyl that had to be accepted back for credit from retail. What's more, consumers accepted prices that allowed a much greater profit margin than LPs. And artists miraculously accepted lower royalties for CDs, thanks to larger "packaging deductions" labels claimed against what they said were much greater manufacturing costs.
>
> On top of it all, the labels could resell everyone the same recordings they already owned. What was not to love? (p. 95)

The promise of these digital versions for fans was that the compact disk opened up new listening possibilities that we'd been missing. The appeal for music companies was that it reduced the costs associated with packaging, shipping, and storing music—compact disks have a smaller footprint and are less easily damaged than vinyl records—and encouraged fans to re-buy their music in the new format (along with new equipment on which to play it). The result, though, was a demonstration that physical media—the liner notes and images and all that was easily copyrightable—are extraneous to the sounds. Once digitized for compact discs, songs are also digitized for any other medium designed to hold data. And any medium designed to transmit data, too. The few years of the original Napster's personal file-sharing existence (1999–2001) proved that both the demand and the technology were far enough along that Apple could introduce iTunes as the savior of an industry shaken by the specter of piracy and lured by the promise that incremental money is better than no money at all.

The reservoir of digitized music has consequences. Kornbluh (2024) posits that "Algorithms are automated procedures for making patterns and exchanges, compositing differing units into higher-order categories. They thus fabricate consistency where there was variability and can effectuate a certain homogeneity: it's all data" (p. 127). And for Fisher (2008/2022), our situation is one in which eclecticism has replaced innovation and collection has become our passion. "Tradition," he maintains, "counts for nothing when it is no longer contested and modified. A culture that is merely preserved is no culture at all" (p. 3).

Fisher rightly calls the good old "new" music a product of a "recombinatorial delirium" (this saves him from the untenable position of arguing for the utter uniqueness of the new). There are easy examples of this. One of the immediate lessons we are taught by the Netflix television series *The Get Down* (2016, an often beautiful example of the commodification of the past via a great, commercial *video* archive) is that hip hop was born as a response to and against the glitz and elitism of disco. And while the argument of the television series may have been simplified for dramatic purposes (it all but omits the foundational radio work of DJ Hollywood, for instance), there's little doubt that the instrumentation of hip hop grew from the techniques DJs developed to extend the drum break, the groove, for the dance floor. And the soul and funk vinyl records that hip-hop DJs inherited from their parents—especially the percussive breaks in those songs—were literally the instruments for what came next. Perhaps every musical scene is defined in part both by its *difference* from what immediately preceded it and by its technical, emotional, and material *debt* to that scene. That is, the new scene is established both differentially and narratively through an established (and establishment) consumer product that becomes a medium.

Jamie Sexton (2012) suggests that this point about debt is increasingly relevant for musicians now, as "contemporary music culture is saturated by artifacts from previous eras. Whilst this has been the case for many years, it is undoubtedly a condition that has increased with the rise of digital technologies and the ability to gain access to a range of recordings and styles from different periods with relative ease" (p. 562). The potentials of music-making equipment available now—to individuals working alone or in small groups in their bedrooms and garages—dwarf those of the best studios of previous decades. In the twenty-first Century, magnetic tape recording radicalized and democratized music making, but not nearly on the scale that digital technologies make possible today. The financial constraints of professional recording studios have loosened and technical knowledge is easily available online. The possibilities for innovation are staggering, but we can also make "new" grunge and hip-hop and punk and disco with an unprecedented degree of accuracy. As musician David Byrne (2017) points out, "Music eats its young and gives birth to a new hybrid creature. I doubt there is a single hip-hop artist whose beats still originate from a DJ manipulating vinyl by hand, but the organizing principal hasn't changed much in thirty years" (p. 119). Neo-folk bands, alternative country, pop punk, and Justin Timberlake[3] are also examples of this kind of new old music, and they are authentic in much the same way that the costumes of period television dramas are.

Fisher (2014) is (probably predictably) bothered by recent appropriations of previous styles separated from their material and cultural pressures:

> Discrepancies in texture—the results of modern studio and recording techniques—mean that they belong neither to the present nor to the past but to some implied 'timeless' era, an eternal 1960s or an eternal 80s. The "classic" sound, its elements now serenely liberated from the pressures of historical becoming, can now be periodically buffed up by new technology. (p. 11)

The new sounds newly old while, through remastering and remixing for digital platforms, the old passes for new.

Broadly, Fisher's assessment rings true, though it also feels very much like a grown-up nostalgically complaining that his music was better than what these damn kids listen to today. Certainly, commercial technology has made songs available in ways they have never been before. Not only is access to vast libraries of music relatively easy for an increasing number of people world-wide, but the actual *material media* by which music has been available—records, cassettes, compact disks—have given way to virtual files that are infinitely copiable and easily distributed. It's possible that what Fisher sees as a breakdown in innovation is, at least partly, the breakdown of legacy media, as radio stations and music critics have lost their tastemaker hegemony and many small, primarily digital communities support cultural productions of all sorts that no longer *need* to break into the larger public arena to be viable.

Even before digital ubiquity, corporate consolidation of radio stations and music companies in the 1980s and 90s—often with parent companies who had no interest in music outside of its revenue-generating

[3] Justin Timberlake returns in the sixth chapter via comics writer Warren Ellis.

potential—meant more attention to the bottom line and less interest in taking risks or nurturing talent. This certainly jibes with Fisher's complaints. But because of the ubiquity of digital production and distribution heralded by Napster and capitalized upon by Apple, costs for production and distribution have maybe lowered to levels that make experimentation more possible than before.

Svetlana Boym (2002) offers a kinder reading than Fisher, offering that, while "nostalgia mourns distances and disjunctures between times and spaces, never bridging them, technology offers solutions and builds bridges, saving the time that the nostalgic loves to waste" (p. 346). It's possible that influences are gathered and remixed in exactly the kind of recombinatorial delirium that Fisher mourns and that there is much innovative, startling work that just cannot now get the critical mass of a zeitgeist. And maybe it doesn't need to. Global markets can make even small niches large enough.

But it's still difficult to dismiss the feeling that there has been a kind of broad stasis in which nostalgia has replaced any excitement about the future. Films are franchises or remakes, and television shows are set in the 1960s or 1980s. A lot of music sounds familiar, and even the supposed avant-garde acts remind us of David Bowie, Alice Cooper, or Menudo.

And, if—to follow Fisher (and Žižek and Jameson)—it's easier to imagine the end of the world than the end of capitalism, then (per the following chapters) it's easier to imagine the world ending than to envision a future very different from now. There was evidence of this back in the 1990s, as the anxiety about the end of history typified by the year 2000 intensified and that decade seemed to stretch. Fredrick Jameson (1996; to whom Fisher acknowledges a great debt) points to the paradox of the post-modern, post-Fordist situation in "the equivalence between an unparalleled rate of change on all the levels of social life and an unparalleled standardization of everything—feelings along with consumer goods, language along with built space—that would seem incompatible with such mutability" (p. 15). In the current age of "disruption," in which every industry (transportation, hotels, education, whatever) should be disrupted because it's possible to do so, and in which this disruption is considered a good by and for itself, change has begun to feel like a constant state. Here, in this "gleaming science-fictional stasis," argues Jameson,

> it is as if the logic of fashion had, accompanying the multifarious penetration of its omnipresent images, begun to bind and identify itself with the social and psychic fabric in some ultimately inextricable way, which tends to make it over into the very logic of our system as a whole. The experience and the value of perpetual change thereby comes to govern language and feelings, fully as much as the buildings and the garments of this particular society, to the point at which even the relative meaning allowed by uneven development (or "nonsynchronous synchronicity") is no longer comprehensible, and the supreme value of the New and of innovation, as both modernism and modernization grasped it, fades away against a steady stream of momentum and variation that at some outer limit seems stable and motionless. (p. 17)

Technological change was certainly accelerating in the 1990s and has reached, now, a state of constancy such that recycling and novelty are consubstantial. Perhaps this late symptom of postmodernity (itself now a nostalgic enterprise) may also be a symptom of late capitalism and the flattening that commodification institutes?

Novelist and design maven Bruce Sterling (2010) has called this stasis *atemporality*, a time *after history* when the world seems to be in stasis, or at least in conservation mode. Less the kitsch that Lyotard describes as the postmodern condition, the current condition promotes niche obsessions more than it does eclecticism. The recent marketing of nerd culture is an example of this (including the fights regarding who gets to be called an authentic nerd, often as a mask for an ingrained sexism), as is the industry of self-publishing and direct sales of music to whatever public has internet access.

To return to the game I played with my students, it may simply be that there has been no Sound of the twenty-first century decades because disintermediation has become our regular state. It's easy now to find people who like what I like without having to be (obviously and broadly) *told* what to like. What some see as the breakdown of novelty could just as easily be its distribution and democratization.

Still, it's weird that even some of the most obscure or niche music available to me when I was in high school is also music some of my undergraduates listened to in high school. I think that they think it's weird, too.

The Tapes of my Youth

When I was a teenager in the 1980s, New Wave or post-punk or whatever we call it now was *my* music, our *authentic* expression. We bought albums and cassettes—and recorded each other's albums onto cassettes, made mixtapes that were "personal"—and dressed as our own approximations of the musicians we saw in music videos, in concert films, and in magazines. In this, we were more or less like the couple of generations (at least) before us. The differences and the rebellion that we performed were little else but a misrecognition of repetition, the repetition of teenage tropes and of whatever marketing reached us. What kept us from recognizing the conformity of our behavior (never mind the later grunge t-shirt and flannel uniformity of the 1990s) was that the difference that counted was only our difference from our parents.

Of course, for a lot of us (usually mostly) white, lower-middle-class kids, at least some of that difference was supported financially *by* our parents, whether they wanted to or not. Often, I'd hoard my school lunch money to buy cassettes. Surely, part of the pleasure that came from my Dead Kennedys collection was that the cassettes were purchased with funds intended for something else. My parents certainly would not have approved of the re-appropriation or the music and, in doing without lunches, I sacrificed a little bit for the fight.

Cassettes were an important medium. If music is a more-or-less traditional means for marking separation from the past, then it is probably not an accident that *the* technology of our autonomy in the 1980s was the cassette-playing Sony Walkman. Introduced widely at the beginning of the decade and almost immediately encouraging cheaper copies (mine was, I think, from Panasonic), the Walkman marked a sonic break from the previous generation with unprecedented precision. Shuhei Hosokawa (2012) argues that the Walkman "represents parasitic and/or symbiotic *self* which has now become autonomous and mobile" (p. 105). Which is to say, not only could my music mark my difference from my parents, but now it could do so outside of my bedroom. The Walkman and other portable cassette players made privacy mobile. To an important degree, anywhere, at any time, I could silence the rest of the sounds of the world in favor of the sounds I chose to hear.

Choice should have been pretty limited for a teenager in a relatively isolated town in West Texas. The shopping-mall record store tended to cater to the broadest market for obvious reasons, and there, those broad tastes ran to country and Top 40. But cassettes also made it easy to copy and disseminate music. The coincidence of a large air force base in town meant an influx of kids from all over the country. They brought their music with them and were happy to share, as long as I sprung for the blank cassettes. My new interests were mostly British post punk, New Wave, and a little California punk, often an album on each side chosen solely to fill holes in my collection, so that certain albums are indelibly tied together because of that accident. For me, Siouxsie and the Banshees' *Join Hands* (1979) and Echo and the Bunnymen's *Heaven Up Here* (1981) were, in 1985, sides A and B of the same listening experience.

While cassettes are durable (they can often be fixed with patience and a pencil), they are only broadly so. Damage in analog is pretty easy to recover from, though. Accidents in recording or tiny injuries to the tape could alter a song forever, at least for its owner, but that damage would become part of the song. A hiccup in my cassette copy of the Talking Heads *Fear of Music* (1979) near the end of the song "Drugs" that I had come to expect didn't make it into the This Mortal Coil cover of the song (on *Filigree & Shadow* 1986), though I would catch myself listening for it.

Even unblemished, the saturation and compression endemic to cassettes lose to the depth of sound possible from vinyl records. And when cassettes are duplicated over and over, sound degrades quickly. These were my first conscious experiences with the maxim *convenience trumps fidelity*. Choosing between having something and having nothing doesn't take much deliberation, especially since, outside of these cassettes or evenings spent listening at friends' houses, I didn't really know what these albums were *supposed* to sound like.

A friend once gave me a copy of a cassette recorded on a boom box backstage by a friend of a roadie at a mid-80 s U2 concert. It was recorded from one side of the stage, the levels were of course terrible, and the tape had been duplicated many, many times. There's no telling which generation I had. But, in a weird perversion of Walter Benjamin's aura of authenticity, the experience of the concert it captured made the cassette valuable, unique, a physical artifact that—much like Plato's metaphor of the transfer of divinity in *Ion*—gained its specialness literally through magnetism.

This isn't to say that fidelity didn't matter to some people. A few friends had access to heavy stereo equipment from the 1960s and 1970s. Their records—mostly country, rock and roll, and jazz—sounded fantastically deep and made listening to music a sit-down, almost worshipful occasion. Probably predictably, with the resurgence of vinyl and the availability of old records just mouse clicks away, some of us have built reminiscent situations out of new and vintage audio equipment. But these living room scenes are always re-creations of poor memories. While buying actual old records can be simple nostalgia plays, buying new work on "old" media may be directly aimed at an almost fetishistic staging of pasts we dimly remember or have only seen pictures of. Dominic Pettman (2017) makes this exact point in *Sonic Intimacy*: "The perfect 'warm' reproduction so coveted by audiophiles from the 1960s through the 1980s is today merely a Platonic ideal, or at best an expensive type of nostalgia." (p. 41). That staging is more likely a staging of fantasy than any reproduction of an actual experience.

Of course, those of us who indulge in building up new systems, like all collectors and investors, recognize that what we enjoy is something that's staged *by* us as much as for us. The entirety of the September 2017 edition of the now-defunct UK music production magazine *Future Music* was dedicated to recapturing the low-fi sounds of the past, either by using modern reproductions of old analog gear or by employing software plugins for digital audio workstations (DAWs) in order to introduce computer-generated tape hiss and vinyl pops to digitally-produced music. "One of the biggest problems with modern instruments and effects," writes the editor in his introduction to the issue, "is that they can sound a little *too* good" (Truss. p. 7). Plugging old instruments into digital audio workstations and using effects to scratch up digital productions seems cynical, but we all know that such music isn't trying to pass as an example of the past, but is participating with it. This knowledge is precisely what, according Žižek,

> renders the fetishist disavowal (split) at its purest—its message is: "I know very well there is no special ingredient, but I nonetheless believe in it (and act accordingly)…" Cynical denunciation (at the level of rational knowledge) is counteracted by a call to "irrational" belief—and this is the most elementary formula of how ideology functions today. ("Hollywood Today: Report from an Ideological Frontline," n.d.)

Treating the past as a special ingredient for new music makes the selection of that ingredient as much a market-driven as an aesthetic choice.

But this more adult participation in the ideology of consumer capitalism was beyond us back then. Where the distance we might be trying to collapse as adults is a temporal one (nostalgia is in this sense a staged intimacy with a fantasy partner; that's why we put on expensive headphones and close our eyes), what we were after in those pre-internet West Texas days was some kind of participation with kids in California or New York or Manchester. And cassettes were our vehicles for crossing to those territories.[4] That cassette tapes hissed and sputtered like the old cars we maybe also got to drive then was only appropriate.

Of course, we could also record our own stuff to cassettes and, while it would be a stretch to claim that this ability spawned a surge in amateur musicianship in my West Texas town, it did produce some experimentation and play that might have never happened otherwise. This was not a new phenomenon. At the beginning of the twentieth Century, very early commercial record players had the ability to record, too. As David Hendy (2013) describes it, "in middle-class homes with a phonograph, people were more likely to record and listen back to their own family members. They would draw the parlour curtains, invite friends around, summon

[4] Recreating the sounds of old media now seems—to me—to lose that feeling of participation, as it refers back to "me back then," not just "back then.".

up the bodiless voices, then hear them float uncannily through the air. It was a kind of séance in which they got to choose their own ghosts" (ch. 25). But music companies eventually realized that they could make more money selling prerecorded disks if folks couldn't make their own. Sony's co-founder Masaru Ibuka seemed to have intuited that in the late 1970s when he proposed removing microphones from cassette players to make them more portable. Walkmans were strictly for consumption.

Regardless of the fidelity or provenance, the transportability of music helped me move my privacy into the public. This is, of course, still the case. As Mark Katz (2010) describes it in *Capturing Sound*,

> solitary listeners are everywhere, both in the privacy of their homes and out in the world. But there is—or at least should be—something strange about seeing people in public places, earphones practically implanted into their brains, nodding or singing along to their own private music. Journalist Paul Fahri wonderfully captured that strangeness, evoking images from the classic horror movie Night of the Living Dead: "It is so familiar now that we don't see or hear it anymore. It is the look and sound of the Walkman dead: the head cocked at a slight angle, the mouth gently lolling. From about the skull comes a tinny low buzzing sound, like metallic bees. The eyes flicker with consciousness, but they don't see. They're somewhere else." Perhaps we should wonder not that solitary listening was once considered unusual but rather that it should have come to be so widely, unremarkably practiced. The same is true for the act of listening to music far removed from one's home or culture or of experiencing music whenever and with whomever one wishes. In each case, the portability of recording has made the once unimaginable commonplace. (p. 21)

The Walkman and its copies allowed the aestheticization of almost any situation. This was a machine that set us free from our bedrooms to wander, zombie-like, to the beat of various drums.

Now, digital formats are much more portable. They take up no physical space at all. And the privatizing of music consumption that cassettes introduced has of course found its zenith in today's digital distribution enterprises, where specific tastes and expectations can be marketed to directly, while algorithms predict what we will have liked.

There has been a material change, too. In an interview with *Wired* magazine in 2004, Michael Bull, author of *Sounding out the City: Personal Stereos and the Management of Everyday Life* (2000), suggests in the context of Apple's then-new iPod mini:

> One of the interesting things is that with vinyl, the aesthetic was in the cover of the record. You had the sleeve, the artwork, the liner notes. With the rise of digital, the aesthetic has left the object—the record sleeve—and now the aesthetic is in the artifact: the iPod, not the music. The aesthetic has moved from the disc to what you play it on … and the iPod mini will appeal to those who want an artifact for style…. ("Bull Session With Professor IPod")

iPods and other players perfected the cassette Walkman by making any music I could get (from my own collection, from friends, from Napster) available on a (then) massive hard drive I could carry around. Playlists replaced albums and mixtapes were easy. These players gave us absolute control.

The iPod mini has since been retired, replaced by phones and other connected devices that have been or are becoming commoditized, losing through their ubiquity the aesthetic aura that those old devices had. And it's more and more likely that the music we access on the go isn't from files we've collected, but from bits streamed through services we subscribe to that offer the current hits we like, but also playlists by taste-makers, cool kids, and algorithms. We are more than happy to give up control for the ease of surprise.

But, as Mark Katz notes, "The Internet not only makes it possible to find particular pieces easily, it also allows users to explore unfamiliar territory. If one can imagine a particular type of music, it probably exists; if it exists, it can probably be found on the Internet" (p. 186). Availability doesn't guarantee exploration and discoveries of new musical interests, of course. I can still choose to listen to what I've always listened to (or have others choose for me).[5] But the vast network of archives available on the

[5] In *A Primer for Forgetting* (2019), Lewis Hyde writes, "Replying to a question about the effort he put into composing with chance operations, John Cage said, 'It's an attempt to open our minds to possibilities other than the ones we remember, and the ones we already know we

internet can serve up the new, or at least the new-to-me. No one needs to rely on adjacent military bases any longer.

It's possible, though, that while accessibility means broader access to niche interests, ubiquity also makes listening less special. Damon Krukowski (2017) laments: "I for one find myself clicking through a good deal of digital music. If it's online or on my computer, I skip around—I preview tracks, hearing a bit here, a bit there" (p. 121). In contrast, Erik Satie was famously upset when people stopped to listen to the "furniture music" he had designed to be background for sociality. In the early 1900s, music in public was rare enough that people treated it with a direct and appreciative attention. The ubiquity of private music in public spaces has now made every piece a potential background for the day, and the shuffling that Krukowski describes is most like searching for the appropriate soundtrack for the present activity.

The ubiquity of music of a relatively even quality opens up access to work that would otherwise be unavailable and underappreciated, makes it respectable, but it can also commodify music to such an extent that what might have made a particular example special—its rarity, its provenance, its aura, whatever—is rendered of even a pretense of its subversive power.

Goth Is a Mall Store

Rebellion and non-conformity are difficult when every passing interest is registered in the databases that track and help serve me advertisements for what I should want. Non-conformity is *fashionable*. And, like all fashion, it is recyclable. Again, Fisher (2008/2022):

like. Something has to be done to get us free of our memories and choices.' Or he once said, 'This is … why it is so difficult to listen to music we are familiar with; memory has acted to keep us aware of what will happen next, and so it is almost impossible to remain alive in the presence of a well-known masterpiece. Now and then it happens, and when it does, it partakes of the miraculous.'" (p. 11).

> Witness, for instance, the establishment of settled "alternative" or "independent" cultural zones, which endlessly repeat older gestures of rebellion and contestation as if for the first time. "Alternative" and "independent" don't designate something outside mainstream culture; rather, they are styles, in fact the dominant styles, within the mainstream. (p. 9)

What was maybe once subversive is now incorporated, stocked on shelves with easy retail availability. This is the mode of late capitalism. For the system of equivalence that reduces everything to a monetary value, *every* position—even those at odds with each other—is a market.

So, is authentic rebellion even possible anymore?

Was it ever? As a teenager back in the 1980s (and now), finding an identity separate from adults was essential. Nothing mattered more. But the only means available to perform that difference was (and is) via establish mainstream social and economic channels. So the goth clothes I tried on for a very brief instant (or the hair perm I had for a week that thankfully there is no existing photographic record of) were always borrowed and were never ever my own. I could only wear and *be* what was available to me. That I approximated looks from television, album covers, and magazines with thrift store finds then and that, nowadays, goth is a mall store marks a difference in real estate and degree, not in kind.

The irony of authenticity is that it's always purchased from others. Nothing is innately authentic. There is no "real me" trying to express itself from the interior.[6] Or, rather, whatever special something rests at my center, it's there as a foreign body. As Slavoj Žižek (1992/2001) argues:

> insisting on a false mask brings us nearer to a true, authentic subjective position than throwing off the mask and displaying our "true face".... A mask is never simply "a mask" since it determines the actual place we occupy in the intersubjective symbolic network; what is effectively false and null is our "inner distance" from the mask we wear (the "social role" we play), our "true self" hidden beneath it. The path to an authentic subjective position runs therefore "from the outside inward": first, we pretend to be something, we just act as if we are that, till, step by step,

[6] More on this from a psychoanalytic direction in the concluding chapters.

> we actually become it.... In other words, the conclusion to be drawn from this dialectic is the exact opposite of the common wisdom by which every human act (achievement, deed) is ultimately just an act (posture, pretense): the only authenticity at our disposal is that of impersonation, of "taking our act (posture) seriously." (p. 33–34)

While building difference or distance between us and adults may have been essential, there is nothing *essential* about what form that difference takes and the costumes we wear are, if not arbitrary, at least contingent. This does not in any way change the fact that these costumes can be very serious.

Popular music seems especially invested in the costumes of authenticity. In the first half of the previous century, John Lomax toured Huddy Ledbetter—Leadbelly—throughout the United States in out-of-date prison uniforms to accent his "authenticity" (though Ledbetter initially preferred suits). An entire chapter of Hugh Barker and Yuval Taylor's *Faking it: the Quest for Authenticity in Popular Music* (2007) is dedicated to the paradox of punk bands' obvious and exaggerated performances (in particular, the Sex Pistols) and the authenticity they were intended to communicate.

Velvet Goldmine (1998), Todd Haynes's fantasy staging of 1970s Glam Rock and its eventual sell-out in the 1980s is introduced, in some ways, as science fiction. Oscar Wilde, the aesthetic father of Glam (we're shown) was left to us in a basket by a spacecraft from another planet. The transgressive beauty of a later barely-disguised David Bowie character is treated as the legacy of an alien—specially gendered—difference injected into this world from elsewhere. One of the arguments of the film is that there was a substantial number of kids who felt alien in the world of their parents, who felt at home in the costumes of glam, and who felt rightfully betrayed by its corporate cooption.

Authentic music is supposed to be transgressive. Its authenticity lies both in its responses to (uses of) what has come (usually immediately) before *and* the denunciation of that predecessor. Again, difference and debt. Punk rejected the excesses of progressive rock while keeping the basic instruments and song structures of the pop music of previous decades. Rap literally scratched soul and disco records.

But music is also an industry, so while authenticity is, at least partly, a *narrative* enterprise, we should probably not ignore the *enterprise* part. It may be that, in our time of the ubiquitous archive, the flattening of data (and music and texts) makes transgression impossible *except* as marketing. As Steven Shaviro (2015) argues:

> Far from being subversive, transgression today is entirely normative.... Every supposedly "transgressive" act or representation expands the field of capital investment. It opens up new territories to appropriate, and jump-starts new processes from which to extract surplus value. What else could happen, at a time when leisure and enjoyment have themselves become forms of labor? Business and marketing practices today are increasingly focused upon novelty and innovation. More rapid turnover is one way to combat what Marx called the tendential fall of the rate of profit. Far from being subversive or oppositional, transgression is the actual motor of capitalist expansion today.... (p. 31–32)

There's nothing to react against or even *for*. Every orientation should be equally available, equally purchasable, and equally new. The gap between the past and present is evacuated—in what Byung-Chul Han (2017) calls "the total memory of the Digital"—as the archive becomes a marketplace (p. 62). And potential to (eventually) subvert is foreclosed as the present becomes a monotony of novelty and capitalist expansion that "seeks to deplete the future in advance" so that every change is already accounted for (Shaviro, 2015, p. 11). Everything feels static as endless innovation becomes a steady state of constant cyclic churning, all pasts are present, and the future is something we have already purchased as a monthly subscription. Authenticity is impossible when both its differential and narrative components are closed off.

But perhaps that has always been the case, and that's why we become nostalgic. I feel nostalgia for a time when the fantasy of authenticity *was* possible, when the past and the future were still discrete and clear.

And fantasy is probably the right word. Svetlana Boym (2002) indicates nostalgia's relationship to the past and the present when she writes that nostalgia "is a longing for a home that no longer exists or has never existed. Nostalgia is a sentiment of loss and displacement, but it is also a romance with one's own fantasy" (15). We feel like we've lost something, but we also *enjoy* that feeling of loss. We may be in love with it. Fantasy is the mechanism by which we enjoy what we don't have now. Fantasy makes up for absence. Fantasy is also a trace or outline of what was lost, whether or not what was lost ever really existed.

If we assume that a genuine, autodidactic authenticity is impossible—and I think we should—then rendering it merely unavailable is a pretty good magic trick. Talking about movies, Todd McGowan (2008) argues that fantasy "allows the subject to relate to the lost object as an object that is simply out of reach. In fantasy, a spatial or temporal barrier, rather than an ontological one, intervenes between the subject and the lost object" (p. 24). If authentic (non-purchasable) authenticity is impossible, then the stories of when it *was* possible are what sustains the myth of authenticity. The heroes and antiheroes of Gangster films and Westerns are ineffably authentic in their natural exceptionalism, often marked by a difference in costume or through a subtle behavioral tic. Or, for a few days, permed hair.

The results of projecting the exceptional or impossible into the past as something we have lost *is* nostalgia. At its worst, nostalgia can be a call to arms to protect an imagined way of life. As Boym (2002) describes:

> Home is not made of individual memories but of collective projections and "rational delusions." Paranoiac reconstruction of home is predicated on the fantasy of persecution. This is not simply "forgetting of reality" but a psychotic substitution of actual experiences with a dark conspiratorial vision: the creation of a delusionary homeland. Tradition in this way is to be restored with a nearly apocalyptic vengeance. (p. 235)

All soft feelings for the old days and feverish Donald-Trumpian calls to "Make America Great Again" rely on the transformation of ontological impossibility into temporal loss and the libidinal enjoyment that misrecognition brings.

But what kind of fantasy is sustained by projecting the missing, impossible object in the opposite direction? Since the future has also been evacuated by the market, can we feel nostalgia for the futures we've lost?

What Will Have Been Cool

Our son Ben and I talk a lot about music. But beyond generational high-school devotions (he digs my Joy Division and Laurie Anderson and I like his Death Grips and Kendrick Lamar), back at the beginning of the second decade of this century we each found ourselves drawn to and sharing music that directly refences pasts we weren't involved in but that nonetheless resonated with us: the British hauntological and the American hypnogogic, respectively. These are genres that feel like nostalgic exercises, but I've never been British and Ben wasn't alive in the 1980s. In relation to this music we've enjoyed, these nostalgias shouldn't be so available to us, right?

In 2009, David Keenan offered the broad, general definition that "Hypnagogic pop is pop music refracted through the memory of a memory," performing the United States of the 1980s and early 90s through a revisionist nostalgia (26). And just a few years earlier, Mark Fisher pasted the Derridean term *hauntology* to a certain kind of music I found myself drawn to that was surfacing in England around the middle part of the first decade of the twenty-first Century, a music that in part gathers up the electronic sounds of pre-Thatcher 1970s British television.

While there are many examples of outright pop that's hypnagogic (Ariel Pink, Pocahaunted), I'm using the term more broadly here to describe the kinds of American music that point back to 1980s' material and sonic extravagances, the *memory of a memory* of what media life was like back then. Ben's favorite flavor was vaporwave and its many descendants, subgenres that find in 1980s excess the roots of globalization and rabid consumerism and then grapple with these sonically, often in slow motion. In his book on vaporwave, *Babbling Corpse*, Grafton Tanner (2016) declares that "an over-arching definition of vaporwave is harmful, for something so compartmentalizing as a 'How-To Guide' for making vaporwave or a one-sentence summation of the genre seems out of step with the anti-corporatism of the vaporwave composers" (ch. 3). That's probably accurate, and I'm certain I can't offer anything definitive here. Broadly, though, this music takes many of its references from the commercial music (and often the sounds of actual commercials) from the 1980s and 90s. Vaporwave music includes slightly slowed pop hits like

Toto's "Africa" (1982) put through a reverb effect, chopped and screwed synthesizer-and-saxophone easy listening originally played through shopping mall speakers, new compositions reminiscent of Japanese City Pop, and a lot more. In almost every case, the music that this music points back to is made of sounds tied to glossy commerce and suburban middle-class monoculture. Scott Beauchamp (2016) suggests that vaporwave music "sort of offers up an alternative history of post-Cold War America" (para. 14). And Spencer Clark, one of the first hypnagogic artists, maintains that "It's more important to say that the patina of different eras is like time travel; to recognise the essence of the past is to imagine the future" (Keenan, p. 26).

We might say, in our best advertising voiceover, The Future is Now.

As is probably proper for my age, my tastes run just slightly more old school. And hauntological music is maybe more easily described. Music by bands on the Ghost Box label—The Advisory Circle, The Focus Group, Belbury Poly, Pye Corner Audio, and others—often takes as its reference the 1960s and 70s, referring especially to music from the 1970s schools' programs and television shows familiar to me from PBS rebroadcasts of *Doctor Who* episodes and wherever I encountered *Children of the Stones* (1976) and *The Tomorrow People* (1973). These new works surface a strange sonic landscape and evoke weird possible worlds that never quite materialized. In Mark Fisher's (2013) words, "[Hauntological] music and covert art constitute an oneiric conflation of weird fiction, the music of the BBC Radiophonic Workshop and the lost public spaces of the so-called postwar consensus (a consensus that was terminated with the election of Margaret Thatcher in 1979)" (p. 45). In every case, the music Fisher points to calls up the past in unsettling ways. The work is haunted by promise, potential, and loss.[7]

Ghosts are promise, potential, and loss.

[7] Robin James (2025, p. 14) points out that Fisher's hauntology doesn't account for much music produced then and since (Black music in the US, for instance), and that his is largely a white, Eurocentric framing. I don't disagree, and the partiality she points to is precisely the importance of the qualifying anecdotal approach here (and in Fisher's work, too). Grace Jones is a perfect example of repetition that registers otherwise. Additionally, the futurism of Detroit's electro act Drexciya also comes to mind, and I can't imagine a better example of recombinatorial delirium than Madlib's 2003 album *Shades of Blue*.

Derrida (1994) first used the term hauntology in *Specters of Marx*, writing: "To haunt does not mean to be present, and it is necessary to introduce haunting into the very construction of a concept. Of every concept, beginning with the concepts of being and time. That is what we would be calling here a hauntology. Ontology opposes it only in a movement of exorcism. Ontology is a conjuration" (p. 202). Something extra is necessary, something introduced from the outside that doesn't get counted. Hauntology designates a spectral surplus of and for being and time. A haunting perhaps indicates an impasse or impossibility that needs accounting for, rendered in the present as an object that is always missing and is conspicuous by or through its absence.

So, should we perhaps imagine nostalgia for something we feel like we lost in the past—or even a generalized feeling of loss—as a kind of haunting of the present by the past? Maybe especially the pasts of our youth, when times were simpler because we were?

Nostalgia can clearly be a cause for action in the present. Calls to make whatever great again or to return to the good old days rely on a certain constituency's nostalgia for some time previous, whether or not that constituency really experienced that time. Or whether or not that time even really existed that way. Svetlana Boym (2002) calls this kind restorative nostalgia, a nostalgia dedicated to the restoration of origins and conspiracy theories driven by "anxiety about those who draw attention to historical incongruities between past and present and thus question the wholeness and continuity of the restored tradition" (p. 44–45). Against this, she offers a reflective nostalgia that "is more concerned with historical and individual time, with the irrevocability of the past and human finitude" (p. 49).

Certainly, the restorative form of nostalgia demonstrates a dissatisfaction with the present. It's why we're looking back. And we can also imagine our dissatisfaction with the present when compared to an imaginary past as a goad toward a more fulfilling future. Such would depend upon seeing the past as a site of what has since been lost and the future as a place where we will have reclaimed what was lost. The past and the future, then, would overlap at the point of *having*, and the present would be defined by *loss*. Restorative nostalgia, and policies that depend upon its deployment, would work toward positivizing a substantive or formal lack, impossibility, warp, impasse, or whatever by making it a *presence* that is *absent now*. In other words, the trick is to demonstrate a contemporary deficiency—prosperity, peace, traditional values, rock and roll—as something we've lost and then promise to get it back. In this way, the past and future are identically full.

A ghost, though, is an *absence* that is present now. A ghost is substantive. A haunting can also be generative, may be a cause, because it also marks a problem with the present. According to Peter Buse and Andrew Stott (1999), in their introduction to *Ghosts: Deconstruction, Psychoanalysis, History*:

> Ghosts arrive from the past and appear in the present. However, the ghost cannot be properly said to belong to the past, even if the apparition represents someone who has been dead for centuries, for the simple reason that a ghost is clearly not the same thing as a person who shares its proper name. Does then the "historical" person who is identified with the ghost properly belong to the present? Surely not, as the idea of a return from death fractures all traditional conceptions of temporality. The temporality to which the ghost is subject is therefore paradoxical, at once they "return" and make their apparitional debut. (p. 11)

Ghosts, then, are always also creatures of the present. We are being haunted *now*. The origin of a haunting may be found in the past—a murder, say—but that cause *as cause* persists as the presence of the departed, as a constant and active returning to what remains of the scene of the crime. A haunting is not a reminder, but the insistence of what has not been—or cannot be— remembered. If I may put on a psychoanalytic hat for a moment (pulled down tight over my ears in the next chapter), as a repetition, a ghost embodies a lack in the record—what Cathy Caruth (1996) calls a latency (p. 17)—that insists as a symptom of what has not been accounted for. A ghost is the return of that which hasn't been counted, in or as a new manifestation, and is thus a fine figure for trauma and its symptom. In any case, in contrast to restorative nostalgic moves, this repetition ties the past *and* future *and present* together in terms of an insisting and insistent lack.

Haunting is not nostalgic. A ghost is what nostalgia is trying to hide.

As a memory of a memory, hypnogogic music figures lack as a double loss, as nostalgia for nostalgia, as the loss of loss that 1980s excess promised and the twenty-first Century internet provides. In *Retromania: Pop's Addiction to its Own Past* (2011), Simon Reynolds argues that these works relate "to cultural memory and the buried utopianism within capitalist commodities, especially those related to consumer technology in the computing and audio-video entertainment area" (p. 81).

Instead of finding its voice in the potential quashed by the enforcement of neoliberal politics of commerce, the hypnagogic works to resurface the gross naiveté and the superficial shimmer of what resulted. Vaporwave often takes up the comfort of sounds and images of 1980s and 90 s advertising, top 40 radio, and computer magazines, processing them even more through effects that emulate tape hiss and vcr tracking problems in order to stage nostalgia, and then loops these to play over and over again. It amplifies, repeats, and thereby aestheticizes the artifacts of a media scene it barely remembers.

Decades ago, Jean-François Lyotard (1984) argued that the modernist aesthetic is nostalgic, allowing "the unpresentable to be put forward only as the missing contents; but the form, because of its recognizable consistency, continues to offer to the reader or viewer matter for solace and pleasure" (p. 81). To the reader and viewer, we might add listener. Formal, generic consistency and comfort are what we enjoy in television, in film, in music, in popular entertainment broadly, as they cover the gaps or suggest a positive, if absent, content that might otherwise be experienced in more traumatic ways.

Genre is a solicitous container. In our recognition of the song as a good representative of the kind of thing it is, we find security. Generic consistency allows us to sing along without ever hearing the words. Which is to say, fantasy is a formal, generic treatment of, or response to, an impossibility or impasse.

Postmodern art, for Lyotard, would be work that "puts forward the unpresentable in the presentation itself," denying the formal comfort of modernism in order to repeat the impossibility of instantiation. The postmodern accommodates the ghostly. The irony is that this accommodation—the acknowledgement of loss as a formative lack or impossibility—treats the future as another case of the past, since the past and present and future all lack in the same way. Where the modernist impulse was to aestheticize whatever and whenever possible, the postmodern impulse was to explore every mode by which we can repeat the impossible.

By preparing a place for what's missing, we can perhaps see where the postmodern and late capitalism overlap. An example is the music streaming archive, discussed above, something like Spotify. Practically speaking, if much of all recorded music is available now, and if older music that has been remastered and digitized for the archive sounds a lot like newer music such that good production only ever means contemporary tastes, then perhaps even nostalgia is becoming impossible. A system without loss—of work or even fidelity—is also a system that lacks nothing. Or, rather, it is a system that has a place always already prepared for everything it lacks *so far*. What it offers is a *lack of lack*, a lack of the possibility of there ever being something not accounted for. And if that something hasn't arrived yet, then for a whole lot of customers, it doesn't exist at all. When music does arrive, there is shelf space awaiting the new addition to the collection once each piece is compiled and compressed into the same packaging. Such is the ordinary psychosis that has become our common state.

It's not an accident that vaporwave has fragmented into a dozen or more morphing sub-sub-genres ("So vaporwave is dead. Long live vaporwave," Beauchamp, para. 5) and that the Ghost Box label has widened its catalog to include new folk and psychpop (though it still describes itself as a "label for a group of artists exploring the misremembered musical history of a parallel world," *Ghost Box*). The moment hauntological and hypnagogic musics were available as playlists, they had to be ditched, not out of some hipsterish impulse to not like what's popular, but because playlists are the emissaries of an archive that cannot permit their kind of substantial lack.

That archive system can, in its own terms, merely perpetuate itself. It is without a future, as the promise and potential of the new are subsumed by the flattening archive and the spirit of marketing. What haunts it is the possibility of substantive, formative lack or impossibility, something that is necessarily excluded, the what-will-have-been of an aborted potential.

In the early 1990s, Slavoj Žižek (1992/2001) suggested:

> Till postmodernism, utopia was an endeavor to break out of the real of historical time into a timeless otherness. With postmodern overlapping of the "end of history" with full disposability of the past in digitalized memory, in this time where we live the atemporal utopia as everyday ideological experience, utopia becomes the longing for the real of history itself, for memory, for the traces of the real past, the attempt to break out of the closed dome into smell and decay of the raw reality. (p. 228)

It seems that to turn to the postmodern is a kind of nostalgia, too. The irony is that the rush to recover and reanimate the past, to remember what it was like and how we enjoyed then, has in effect aestheticized the past. And if we have lost the "smell and decay of raw reality" and a market exists for such odors, there's little doubt that these can be packaged and sold, as well.

Thinking through Boym's distinctions, Lewis Hyde (2019) offers:

> Reflective nostalgia…may dream of an end to exile, but knowing that the home is in ruins and return impossible, it keeps delaying its departure. Yes, it longs to go back, but the stress falls on the longing, not on the home. It has learned to find pleasure in the marks that time leaves on all things—the patina on the bronzes, the candle soot on the frescoes. It has little story to tell going forward, past loss having made it clear that the future is various and unknown. (p. 118)

The types of music that Ben and I have enjoyed together and separately "find pleasure in the marks that time leaves on all things." What we enjoy isn't the lost thing—it was never ours—but the repetition of longing ultimately for a future that can escape with us, a future that will have been cool.

References

Beauchamp, S. (2016, August 18). How vaporwave was created then destroyed by the internet. *Esquire.* https://www.esquire.com/entertainment/music/a47793/what-happened-to-vaporwave/.

Boym, S. (2002). *The future of nostalgia.* Basic Books.

Buse, P., & Stott, A. (Eds.). (1999). *Ghosts: Deconstruction, psychoanalysis, history* (1999 ed.). Palgrave Macmillan.

Brousse, M.-H. (2013). "Ordinary Psychosis in the Light of Lacan's Theory of Discourse." The Psychoanalytical Notebooks of the London Society, (26).

Byrne, D. (2017). How Music Works (Reprint edition). Three Rivers Press.

Caruth, C. (1996). *Unclaimed experience: Trauma, Narrative and History.* Johns Hopkins University Press.

Cohen, E. E. (1945, January 7). A 'teen-age bill of rights; here is a ten-point charter framed to meet the problems of growing youth. *The New York Times.* https://www.nytimes.com/1945/01/07/archives/a-teenage-bill-of-rights-here-is-a-tenpoint-charter-framed-to-meet.html

Derrida, J. (1994). *Specters of Marx: The state of the debt, the work of mourning, and the new international.* Psychology Press.

Fisher, M. (2009). *Capitalist realism: Is there no alternative?* Zero Books.

Fisher, M. (2013). The metaphysics of crackle: Afrofuturism and Hauntology. *Dancecult: Journal of electronic dance music Culture, 5*(2), 42–55.

Fisher, M. (2014). *Ghosts of My Life: Writings on Depression, Hauntology and Lost Futures.* Zero Books.

Fisher, M. (2022). *Ghosts of my life: Writings on depression, Hauntology and lost futures* (2nd ed.). Zero Books.

Ghost Box—About & Contact. (n.d.). Retrieved October 12, 2024, from https://www.ghostbox.co.uk/about-contact

Han, B.-C. (2017). *Psychopolitics: Neoliberalism and new Technologies of Power* (E. Butler, Trans.). Verso.

Hendy, D. (2013). *Noise: A Human History of Sound and Listening* (First Edition). Ecco Press.

Hosokawa, S. (2012). The Walkman effect. In J. Sterne (Ed.), *The sound studies reader* (pp. 104–116). Routledge.

Hyde, L. (2019). *A primer for forgetting: Getting past the past* (Illustrated ed.). Farrar, Straus and Giroux.

James, R. (2025, November). Against the grain: What's wrong with hauntology? *The wire magazine—Adventures in. Modern Music, 501,* 14.

Jameson, F. (1996). *The seeds of time*. Columbia University Press.
Katz, M. (2010). *Capturing sound: How technology has changed music*. University of California Press.
Keenan, D. (2009). Childhood's end. *The Wire, 306*, 26–31.
Kornbluh, A. (2024). *Immediacy: Or, the style of too late capitalism.* Verso.
Krukowski, D. (2017). *The new analog: Listening and reconnecting in a digital world*. The New Press.
Lyotard, J.-F. (1984). *The postmodern condition: A report on knowledge* (G. Bennington & B. Massumi, Trans.). University Of Minnesota Press.
McGowan, T. (2008). *The real gaze: Film theory after Lacan.* State University of New York Press.
Pettman, D. (2017). *Sonic intimacy: Voice, species, Technics.* Stanford University Press.
Reynolds, S. (2011). *Retromania: Pop culture's addiction to its own past*. Farrar, Straus and Giroux.
Richardson, T. (2022). What will have been cool: Notes on Hauntological and hypnogogic music. *Enculturation.* https://www.enculturation.net/what_will_have_been_cool
Sexton, J. (2012). Weird Britain in exile: Ghost box, Hauntology, and alternative heritage. *Popular Music and Society, 35*(4), 561–584.
Shaviro, S. (2015). *No speed limit: Three essays on accelerationism.* University of Minnesota Press.
Sterling, B. (2010, February 10). Atemporality for the creative artist. *Wired*. https://www.wired.com/2010/02/atemporality-for-the-creative-artist/
Tanner, G. (2016). *Babbling corpse: Vaporwave and the commodification of ghosts.* Zero Books.
Taylor, T. D., Katz, M., & Grajeda, T. (Eds.). (2012). *Music, sound, and Technology in America: A documentary history of early phonograph, cinema, and radio* (1st Paperback ed.). Duke University Press Books.
Toop, D. (1995). *Ocean of sound: Ambient sound and radical listening in the age of communication.* Serpent's Tail.
Truss, S. (2017, September). Rough and ready. *Future Music, 331*, 7.
WIRED. (2004, February 25). Bull session with professor IPod. *Wired*. https://www.wired.com/2004/02/bull-session-with-professor-ipod/
Žižek, S. (2001). *Enjoy your symptom!: Jacques Lacan in Hollywood and out* (2nd ed.). Routledge.
Žižek, S. (n.d.). Hollywood today: Report from an ideological frontline. Lacan.Com. Retrieved June 16, 2020, from https://www.lacan.com/essays/?page_id=347

3

All Our Yesterdays

In the third season episode of the original *Star Trek* series titled "All Our Yesterdays" (1969), Kirk, Spock, and McCoy beam down to a planet about to be destroyed by its sun. That is, since all the inhabitants seem to be gone from the planet, they beam down to the *library* of the planet to find out what's happened to the people before the exploding star destroys any record.

In this library, they find a vast archive that, instead of books or films about the histories and cultures of the planet's inhabitants, offers *direct windows* to every moment in the past of the planet and its people. By placing a round disk about the size of a coffee can lid onto a stand (this is a future civilization that still uses physical media; it's alien), the disk becomes a viewscreen through which a patron can see and hear the actual past that disk stands for.

Accidentally, the three men discover that these windows are also doors and that, in order to escape impending doom, all of the people of the

---

Early versions of some parts of this chapter previously appeared in Richardson, T. (2021). Home Bodies: Prosthetic People and Economies of Desire. In C. Neill (Ed.), *Lacanian Perspectives on Blade Runner 2049*, Springer International Publishing, 103–119.

T. Richardson, *Nostalgia, Fantasy, and the Futures of Masculinity*, The Palgrave Lacan Series, https://doi.org/10.1007/978-3-032-23921-1_3

planet—except for one last heroic librarian named Atoz (A to Z!)—have retreated to various moments in their history. Captain Kirk hears a woman scream, runs through a nearby doorway, and ends up in their version of the seventeenth Century. He is quickly accused of witchcraft and imprisoned. McCoy and Spock chase after him, but find themselves in an ice age in which Spock kisses Mariette Hartley. The rest of the episode is spent pulling Kirk back to the library, then Kirk working with the anxious Atoz to get McCoy and Spock back to the present before the planet is destroyed.

The great, mostly empty library is a conceit that allows for the action and is really incidental to the plot. We only see a couple of pretty sparse rooms of what we are left to imagine is a truly huge complex. There could be other ways to get them into similar situations (every offering in the *Star Trek* franchise has been fond of theme planets, for instance). This episode isn't about the library or the planet's inhabitants, but about what happens to and with our heroes after they rush headlong into the unknown to help. That's how these kinds of episodic television shows work: here is a novel situation; what are its repercussions? Variety in these episodes is mostly only an attempt to hide the formula a little bit. In science fiction television, the "science fiction" element is accepted, simply assumed as a catalyst for human action. It has to be. Doors open by themselves. Computers talk. Difference is normalized. Explaining these everyday mysteries would distract from the exciting events of the episode.

When I was a kid watching these in syndication, I wanted to wander around that library, and the fact that it was *just* a narrative device was frustrating. After a little time in what should be an amazing discovery (the ticking-clock exploding star helps explain that little time), the story is left with costuming the seventeenth-Century characters more-or-less appropriately for 1960s television budgets so that they can convincingly worry about witches. An ice age can get by with fur blankets and fantasy loincloths.

Part of the reason I remember it is no doubt because Spock kisses Mariette Hartley. But mostly it felt like a missed opportunity. A conventional, "historical" past played out on an "alien" world makes sense in the character-in-peril plot that most of the episodes follow, but I wanted something else. The plot promised thrills, but the premise offered *wonder*. What is a world with this technology like? Before they knew that they were going to blow up, how did the folks of this planet use the library? Were there only nonfiction works there, or was there room for fiction? If there was fiction, was any of it science fiction, or was this a culture whose curiosity was only backward-looking, nostalgia made literal? How did the librarians even organize this great archive so that all time remained available? Were boring or less useful pasts put in storage? Was there a Special Collections? None of these questions makes good television. All of these questions stuck with me.

Where Saturday morning public service announcements between cartoons had told me to read a book and turn on the tv in my head, this library on television certainly upped the ante. Here, everything everywhen was available *right now*. Once you're able to look in on any moment of history, the past becomes consumable. As with the archives of the previous chapter, in this library, all of the past was *present*. At the end of history, it's only fitting that the final consumer product is being able to participate in your own past, to *be* your own antecedent.

This chapter takes up issues of haunting and repetition in relation to the vast and pervasive present by extending the discussion into other popular culture properties and structures of capitalism through an explicitly psychoanalytic lens. Here, the focus is fantasy (by at least two definitions).

Fantasy Pasts

As "All Our Yesterdays" and any number of other episodes demonstrate, *Star Trek* is as often fantasy television as it is science fiction. Technobabble aside, the magic of mind melds, beaming down, and time travel are as much a part of the series as the science fiction infrastructure of automatic doors, talking computers, and automat-style food replicators.

This isn't very surprising. Until maybe as late as the first decade of the twenty-first century—as nerd culture spread its wings to both hoard and meticulously count and sort its gold—science fiction and fantasy were frequently mixed together in book and video stores sections. And those of us—in the popular imagination, always boys—who enjoyed science fiction and fantasy were thought of, decades before, as likeminded loners who hid in basements playing board games with their weird friends. One of the great business insights of the 1980s and 1990s was that we also had some money available to us. We might have been different from the good folks who enjoyed drama and romance and even action, but it was a difference that could be marketed to.

It still is. We now think nostalgically about those nerd days. The Netflix series *Stranger Things* (2016) is pretty good evidence, as is the explosion of toy collecting and comic book interest since at least the beginning of this century.

Genre work is readily marketable because viewers or readers already have a sense of whether they're going to like whatever that particular work is, based on experience with other things like it. And back then, there wasn't a lot to consume, so we took what we were given. That isn't the case anymore.

Not just the obvious *Lord of the* Rings films, but vampires and zombies and every superhero franchise demonstrate that fantasy has been and remains a very popular genre. The *Bedford Glossary of Literary Terms* (2008) defines *fantasy fiction* as "A type of fiction set wholly or in part in a vaguely medieval Arthurian or imaginary land populated by inhabitants subject to magic, as well as magical figures, creatures, or beasts" (p. 165). The Arthurian bit is maybe a little precious (and may be simply a way to avoid saying Tolkienesque?), but for a brief description, it's a good stab. Fantasy means a long time ago, plus magic. It is often pitched as a non- or a-historical past ("historical" pasts on a made-up *Star Trek* planet also count as fantasy, since they are always modeled on our own imagined histories plus nose prosthetics). These stories tend to work well with swords and leaky roofs; they are more personal, local, and promise close-quarter adventure. And it's fun to watch a pretend, impossible past play out in the present, especially at its most detailed and authentic.

But *magical past* seems pretty limiting for the genre. The *Bedford* entry goes on to maintain that "[a]ttempts to define the term more broadly are complicated by the overlap between fantasy fiction and other genres, such as science fiction and horror, and further compounded by the tendency of fantasy authors to import and mix elements of different genres." Brands aren't always effective in keeping cattle separated. Fencing genres is hard.

Along with horror, sci-fi and fantasy depend to various extents on mostly "impossible" differences from my "real" world and thereby offer eccentric options to daily life. Because of this otherness, Ramzi Fawaz (2011) calls these works Popular Fantasy as a way to discuss very different kinds of impossibilities without having to snip through literary genre fencing (pp. 356, 358). With this, Fawaz participates in a long-running conversation about the fantastic in literature (for him, X-Men comics) as gaps into which theoretical wedges may find purchase. The otherness of Popular Fantasy perhaps draws attention to the contingency of "real world" particulars that might otherwise go unnoticed. It also makes room for fantasies that aren't *historical* but that nonetheless depend on magic (urban fantasies like Laurell Hamilton's *Anita Blake* series and Lev Grossman's *The Magicians*, for instance, or *Buffy the Vampire Slayer*) and the impossibilities of much science fiction.

But it's sometimes useful to narrow definitions. If fantasy is *something*, it should be possible to distinguish that thing from other things like it. Toward this end, but without limiting subject matter too much, Mark Bould (2002) suggests the following:

> Where fantasy differs from other forms of fiction is in the particular nature of its world-building. All fiction builds worlds which are not true to the extratextual world (itself an ideological—and, arguably, therefore a fantastic—construct), but fantasy worlds are constructed upon a more elaborate predicate: they are not only not true to the extratextual world but, by definition, *do not seek or pretend to be*. Recognising its status, fantasy disavows the very possibility of a territory which is not its map.
>
> This concern with world-building, with the paranoid construction of textual ontologies, is consistently foregrounded in fantasy and the fantastic genres. (p. 81, my emphasis)

His points are doubled. First, the self-reflexive, knowing way fantasies build their worlds identifies the commonality of these texts as they are, he goes on to argue, "subsumed into the capitalist culture industry and reified in a commodity form." It's *world-building* that they're *selling*.[1] Each remarkable difference from the real world is possibly a marketable difference, too. The second point is that the meticulous, knowing, and *paranoid* manner in which every element of the world is connected to every other element is what allows that world's packaging and its elaborations into franchises across media. For instance, the same story bible should be consulted for the film, television, and novelized versions of a property, the minutia of which is likely enjoyed by fans as evidence of the authenticity both of a particular version in a given medium and of the fan who enjoys it. What fantasy foregrounds, then, isn't truth, but authenticity.

Authenticity is complicated. Early in "The Work of Art in the Age of Mechanical Reproduction," Walter Benjamin (1969) claims: "The presence of the original is the prerequisite to the concept of authenticity" (p. 220). He then beautifully describes the mechanisms by which the cultic value of a singular work of art is superseded by the ubiquity and accessibility of copies, and then the moment in which there is no longer a question of the original. Photographic prints have no real, enjoyable original. And today's digital artifacts are infinitely copiable and infinitely distributable. Perhaps outside of the act of making, today it's very difficult to christen anything as the original.

Even in the "first" sense of the presence of the original, though, realism and authenticity only truly matter once a copy is introduced against which I can compare it. If there is a question about the authenticity of, say, a painting, investigators will look for clues, differences, anachronisms that could distinguish the original from its copy. In strictly technical terms, a very fine forgery may be much more sophisticated than the original. Benjamin describes this history of authenticity as a move from poor-quality manual reproduction to highly advanced technical (mechanical) reproduction which, he says, "emancipates the work

[1] As much as the early part of this chapter seems to denigrate fantasy for the sake of promoting the presumably (per Darko Suvin and others) more "rational" and "cognitive" science fiction, I am wholly in agreement with China Miéville (2009), that "To the extent that SF claims to be based on 'science', and indeed on what is deemed 'rationality', it is based on capitalist modernity's ideologically projected self-justification: not some abstract/ideal 'science', but capitalist science's bullshit about itself" (p. 240).

of art from its parasitical dependence on ritual"(224). The iterability of a work releases that work from its cultic value and secularizes it. Specialness isn't defined by the unique artifact in its place and time, but by the new contexts (or collections) that *my instance* of the artifact can be situated within. In this way, ritual bends to commodity.

But even after the death of the original, perhaps authenticity remains an issue, if only in a more general or vulgar sense? Authenticity is just as important when we make copies without trying to hide them. Costuming and set design in television shows and movies aren't meant to trick me into thinking that my television, computer, and phone screens are actual windows to the past. And fans dressing up at a comic book convention rarely trick me into believing that I'm seeing Batman in the flesh. In both world-building and fandom, authenticity is a kind of investment in iteration as a performance that is never intended to be confused with "real life."

This kind of authentic performance is trying to convince me of something: that it's okay to pretend, that pretending is serious and useful. And that pretending takes work. Sigmund Freud explored the earnestness of play for children early in "Creative Writers and Daydreaming" to somehow account for the intellectual work of imagining that adults do, sometimes professionally. Kids know very well that what they're doing isn't *real life*, he argued, but that fact doesn't take away the seriousness of what they're playing at. The point of pretending is to explore the rules of the world and to discover which, if any, are arbitrary. For these explorations, fingers can be guns, and so can sticks.

Contrast this with some versions of adult play in which props are almost *required* to be elaborate. The relatively recent rise in popularity of costume play (cosplay) and prop weapons displays is a good example of this, as is the usually fantasy-inflected practice of Live Action Role-Playing (LARPing). These all take significant time, money, or both. The accuracy and realism of props and costumes don't make the practice seem less like play. Props, costumes, and time are *investments* in play, but in a sanctioned, useful, social playing that relies on a shared notion of authenticity.

The insistence on authenticity isn't only the purview of nerd culture. Nothing seems more important to some Civil War reenactors (historical

LARPers) than accuracy and realism, even though—unlike the actual Civil War—everyone gets to go safely home to their families after the battle. It may in fact be that the whole "fun" of this kind of authenticity is participation in an authentically staged scenario that creates a credible world that one *knows* is fake but that is also (or therefore) engaging. Fantasy is self-conscious world-building but, especially in this case, fantasy play intersects with celebrating through the repetition of a certain received heritage.

Participation in something shared and valued is what's important here. Gregory Hall (2015) maintains that the version of the Civil War that is reenacted "is more centered on patriotism and what it means to be American rather than on warfare itself. The battle reenactments themselves are composites of reality and fiction and authenticity is negotiated by the reenactors within shared historical assumptions" (p. 415). The content of what's performed extends beyond the mere repetitions of historical fact and is steeped in common values, one of which is participation in the shared contemporary community. Hall argues that the product of reenactment, the battle, is an excuse for a deeper, more authentic relationship that participants have with a culture and world that they re-inscribe for themselves in the present. Reenactments "are a common sense repetition of cultural norms and expectations.... Maintaining a place in a segment or segments of society requires the processes and products to be understood as authentic and relevant to the present cultural context" (p. 417). The repetition of these norms and expectations is, regardless of the provenance of the accoutrements, bordering on ritual, insofar as repeated performances conjure a space here and now in which the past as a particular, static, authentic manifestation of cultural beliefs and practices can find a home.

As repetition and ritual, it's important to note two things. In *A Rhetoric of Motives*, Kenneth Burke (1969b) argues that ritualized behavior is "a symbolic getting, not a real one. Hence, it could exist only by prolonging or delaying the act.... All purely ritual getting is also a not-getting" (p. 273). Ritual, as a way of ostensibly participating with the past, is also a way in which the present can be projected into the future in a kind of infinite delay. The job of ritual is precisely to render an event repeatable for yourself and for others and at the same time yet-to-come (immanent) by making that event partial and incomplete. But ritualized repetition also works on the past. While repetition imagines an "authentic" origin that *causes* the repetition (we repeat in order to remember something), in actuality the ritualized repetition as a theatrical version of the event is what introduces questions of authenticity into the content. Just like an original painting may gain value because it is copied, an event in the past becomes foundational because it is repeated. In essence, this kind of repetition evacuates the past event of its historical discreteness in order to conjure its presence now and keep it present as *heritage*, as what I carry with me. At the same time, as Burke describes, ritual projects this unsatisfied (perhaps undead) status quo into the future, thus rendering the future *as* the present and depleting it of any radical potential. Repetition is always about the present, and is thereby *for itself*. As Alenka Zupančič (2008) puts it:

> For it seems that there is an inherently theatrical element involved in repetition—theatrical in the sense of belonging to theater, not in the sense of being melodramatic, exaggerated, or affected. This might be explained, at least to some extent, by the point made above: that repetition is essentially repetition of a configuration; that it doesn't represent anything, but is itself the very content of what it represents. (p. 171)

Repetition is like theater, costumes and all. If I were to undertake an analysis of Civil War re-enactment, for instance, then harping on the *authenticity* of the re-enactments would be a mistake. The question to ask isn't *Is this really what it was like?* but *What work is this doing for those involved right now?* The exact same question could be asked about cosplaying at comics conventions, or the recounting of a dream in a psychoanalytic session.

Such conjuring of the past into the present to enjoy is a sign of nostalgia, surely. It is, as Dennis Hall (2004) argues, "an exercise of the nostalgic impulse especially well-suited to the social, political, and economic turmoil of late capitalism," and may be an exercise in the "denial both of the present and of the present's vision of the future" (p. 9). Nostalgia is a common reaction to the complexities of the present. We may be nostalgic for a certain received version of a "historic" past—like some Civil War reenactors and historical society members—or a time much more recent.

The common understanding is that we are often nostalgic for the decades in which we were children and young adults because life seemed less complicated then *for us*, not because the world was a less complicated place for everyone. For many of us, when we were young, the world was smaller, more homogenous, and was determined by rules that seemed static because these rules had existed since we were born (never mind that some of those rules existed *because* we were born). It shouldn't be a surprise, then, that cultural reenactments like cosplay at comic conventions, the conventions themselves, and the game/film/television properties they often celebrate have become bigger and more mainstream. Nerd culture is very much like the Civil-War-reenactor culture that predates it by only a few decades in its allegiance to authenticity, in its gestures to larger and shared cultural assumptions, and in rituals of conserving the shared past it both creates and sustains into adulthood. But what shouldn't be missed here is that what the past was actually like has little bearing on the performance of it now. What is being repeated isn't the past, but iterations of stasis and safety to bolster a fantasy of the past. In contrast to the exploratory play of children, adult play is often definitively conservative.

Fantasy and Fantasy

The cultural assumptions—historic, literary, or filmic—around which groups coalesce can easily become a dogma that needs protection. At the same time, the props and worlds that support these assumptions are commodified as fans and believers occupy the same kind of market. While invented, the elaborate fantasy worlds *matter* to those of us who live in them beyond ways to waste an afternoon. This is as true for *Star Wars* fans as it is for Civil War re-enactors. Complaints about female leads, Black Stormtroopers, and Disney woke-ness in the *Star Wars* franchise indicate, if not a sexism and racism that had been endemic to the franchise, at least major discomfort experienced by some fans with any obvious or perceived change, even as these fans clamor for more episodes.

Fantasy, by its nature, is conservative and iterative. Fantasy is invested in keeping the world a coherent, closed system of intricately networked actants and in policing the boundary for intruders.

In its missions to conserve and to maintain coherence, fantasy as a genre overlaps with the kind of "private" fantasy that's an object of psychoanalytic study. It isn't a stretch to imagine that Todd McGowan (2007) is also describing the completionism of genre-fantasy world building (and Civil War reenactment) when he claims that, within a Lacanian psychoanalytic framework,

> fantasy is an imaginary scenario that fills in the gaps within ideology. In other words, it serves as a way for the individual subject to imagine a path out of the dissatisfaction produced by the demands of social existence.... By distorting social reality through an imaginative act, fantasy creates an opening to the impossible object and thereby allows the subject to glimpse an otherwise inaccessible enjoyment. (p. 23)

Just as manic attention to trivial detail demonstrates the amount of my investment in the wholeness of a fantasy world, my investment in the psychoanalytic brand of fantasy works to "fill the gaps" in the ideological framework of the social "real" world. Both kinds of fantasy are dedicated to maintaining appearances and to the enjoyment I get from that work. Additionally, just as an individual cosplayer at a convention recreates or riffs on an existing commercial property (and so eagerly volunteers to advertise for that property), private fantasies are made up of only what's socially—and often commercially available that can be put to work to sustain a consistency of and in the "real" world (in order to allow me to be a functioning, consuming citizen of it).[2] With both kinds of fantasy, following Bould (2002), "the subject is involved in the practice of making do with the texts and commodities that the apparatus provides" (p. 74). That the genre-related fantasy is more obviously *put on* makes it only slightly easier to market to.

In any case, for genre fantasy, building a sustained and convincing world is important. The opening credits of the television series *Game*

[2] Subsequent chapters will discuss fantasy and markets at length, especially the sixth chapter's examination of RealDolls and Reborns.

of Thrones show viewers an animated map of the world in which the series takes place, giving a crib of the political landscape via the division of lands and indicating in which regions the action of a particular episode will take place. In this, the series mimics the frontispiece of many fantasy books, which include maps showing us readers where we're going in the mythical land and, sometimes, long genealogies or family trees as maps of time. These allow a wide view of the world and its history while simultaneously situating the current action of particular characters in that broader context.

World building is important because often, in these works, the *whole world* has to be rescued from some ancient, dark invading force (winter, we are told, is coming). The world will be saved, of course, by heroes. Frequently, what these hero characters—often youngsters or hayseeds without a lot of world experience—want is for the world they live in to remain predictable enough that they can maintain a home in their simple version of it. Or sometimes their arc is to discover that the world isn't so simple and that they were born into a destiny they can't escape. But then that destiny is simple, though it may only be revealed after a lot of complicated plotting. Again, fantasy is conservative. It's about the rules and kinship and races and politics that engender a world, that make it real. And it's about *saving* the world. That ancient forest is important. Nothing is sadder than elves having to leave their homes forever.

In a note to a brief discussion of the nostalgia and moralism of Tolkienesque fantasy narratives, Bould (2002) makes a similar point:

> A typical narrative of Big Commercial Fantasies, such as David Eddings *Belgariad* (1982–5) series, Raymond Feist's *Riftwar Saga* (1982–92) or *Star Wars* (Lucas, 1977) and its sequels/prequels, features a boy who rises from the ranks of slave, servant or freeman to become a king or powerful wizard who replaces despots without affecting the social order: the ugly duckling follows an Horatio Alger narrative transformed, courtesy of prophecies and fate, into a fantasy of obedience. (p. 58)

Here we could add the Harry Potter books and films, as well as host of other young adult fare. The closed system of fantasy narratives allows for the myth of personal growth without the dangerous unpredictability of (much) social change.[3] The promise is excitement and adventure and a coherent, rigid scaffolding to which I can pledge allegiance. We must save Hogwarts and restore balance to the Force.

The private fantasy of psychoanalytic investigation is also primarily fantasy of and for obedience; fantasy allows a minimal enjoyment as an investment in maintaining the status quo by spackling the gaps with available ideology. For a while now, that ideology has been that of rugged individualism and personal responsibility. The Marlboro Man used to be the literal poster for an ideal that has mutated and is now maintained by calls to "authentic" living via returns to mindfulness, simple and rustic "van life," et cetera, where my life is also my job. In every iteration, these promise personal fulfillment detached from the social, political, and economic systems in which we are emmeshed, while deferring that fulfillment indefinitely, since the versions we see on social media are fantastic and we can only ever fail to live up to them.

But are the pleasures of staging the future the same as those of staging the past? Sometimes, surely. That's space opera, *Flash Gordon* and *Star Wars* and the like. These take the narrative models of popular fantasy—the mythological and magical, but also the tropey predictability—and imagine them in a universe set some time and space away from our own. *Star Wars* takes place a long time ago and is about a young hayseed discovering that he has a destiny. One reason the mention of midichlorians in the first *Star Wars* prequel, *The Phantom Menace* (1999), rankled so many fans is that they recognized someone trying to wedge in a science-fiction normalizing for fantasy magic.

We can, I think, see the witchy and chilly pasts of *Star Trek*'s "All Our Yesterdays" as common costumed fantasies in the long tradition of film and the shorter one of television. But that library makes it science fiction. In the late 1960s, Arthur C. Clarke posited that any "sufficiently advanced technology is indistinguishable from magic" (Clarke 255). A significant number of *Star Trek* episodes ("The Return of the Archons," "The Paradise Syndrome," "For the World Is Hollow and I Have Touched the Sky," etc.) are devoted to unsophisticated aliens believing

[3] The final chapter will discuss in more detail our emphasis on the personal over the systemic.

in the gods that are eventually revealed to be (usually broken) technologies. But really, transporters are technological magic, too. Clarke was one of those very influential Golden Age science fiction authors who—along with Asimov, Heinlein, Bradbury, Pohl, and others— emphasized the genre's ties to what Sherryl Vint (2014) succinctly calls "scientific extrapolation and rationalist logic" (p. 2). The idea was to stress the *science* of the fiction as distinct from fantasy and to illustrate a line from here to there.

The problem is that this doesn't help distinguish fantasy from science fiction, but only excuses some of science fiction's most outlandish extrapolations. If something looks indistinguishable from magic, it isn't recognizably an extrapolation from something familiar. People have to travel from one point to another in space, so I *guess* a transporter that allows you to vanish from one place and appear in another is a kind of extrapolation. But that's really stretching the idea and feels more like an excuse (for cost-effective television in a predestined time slot) than rigorous scientific projection into the future. Rather, a truly speculative science fiction element would take up mundane, unremarkable infrastructure. Steven Shaviro (2024) makes this distinction early in *Fluid Futures: Science Fiction and Potentialities*: "A science-fictional world generally postdates, extends beyond, and departs from—but therefore, to a certain extent, also arises out of—the actual world in which it is written and read" (p. 7). Just like the talking computers in our pockets and automatic doors at the grocery store, what saves the Star Trek library from being pure magical flourish, *only* an enchanted plot device to get our characters from the future to a past, is that it resembles (in concept, if not in presentation) libraries that we know. That library is an amplification of what we had in the 1960s, and resonates with us even more in this age of the ubiquitous digital archive.

Unlike much fantasy, which is often about preventing or recovering from some catastrophic change, the kind of speculative science fiction I'm interested in *presumes* change. It draws attention to even the tiniest differences between our world and its world and keeps prodding. Difference isn't something that heroes resist mightily in service to the plot, but what *insists* regardless of the story, in the background. Doors open by themselves and computers talk to us.

It should be clear that, with the terms speculative and science fiction, I mean something less versatile than Donna Haraway's (2016) *SF*. For her, SF is a term that shifts among "science fiction, speculative feminism, science fantasy, speculative fabulation, science fact, and also, string figures" (10). My use is both broader and more modest. Where Haraway deploys her term to mark potential sites of intervention, I most simply mean the potential to intervene at all, given an ideological framework that seems unshakeable. My argument is maybe closest to what she claims in a note, citing Joshua LaBare, "that sf is not fundamentally a genre," but is rather "a mode of attention" (p. 213). In my estimation, speculation is the potential within any genre to work against the rules or expectations of that genre or, if not actively work against them, to simply *be otherwise*. Speculation marks the foreign element at the center of any ideology.[4]

As an aspect of narrative storytelling, speculation insists on remaining connected with our own experiences through a kind of proximity and dissonance with them. Speculation is about exposing the most minimal of gaps or cuts. It shares its goals with what Wordsworth wanted from poetry: the ability to find similarities in things that we imagine are dissimilar and significant difference in those things we tend to lump together. Both are about estrangement and the best have as their founding mechanism a workaday version of what Freud called *unheimlich*, the unhomely or uncanny.[5]

It isn't difficult to find this same speculative insistence beyond vulgar technologies. Examples are obvious. Gender is defamiliarized in works of Ursula K. Le Guin and Margaret Attwood, as is race in many of Octavia E. Butler's novels and the environment in books by Paolo Bacigalupi

[4] I had thought here about replacing "speculative" with "constructivist," after the old Russian art movement, which had as a central tenant a practicality that's appealing. And constructivist-influenced film directors like Sergei Eisenstein perfected an editing technique that drew attention to the ways in which editing yields an ideological coherence via actual cuts that should normally be all but invisible to an audience when deployed less aggressively, in work that relies of the comforts of easy coherence. Unfortunately, there is a lot of other ideological baggage with that word that makes it less agile. In any case, subsequent chapters discuss the foreignness at the center.

[5] Here, speculative science fiction shares more with the horror genre than with fantasy; much science fiction and horror are both about the strange within the familiar, a crack in the present same- and tameness.

and Cixin Liu. In these cases (and many others), the strange or alien functions to open up a critical gap so that our own overriding anxieties may be amplified safely and palatably. As Vint (2014, glossing Darko Suvin's understanding) explains, such science fiction

> forces us to confront ideas and conventions that have been *made to appear* natural and inevitable, by giving us a world founded on other premises. The dialectical interaction between what is familiar and what is alien thus opens up a more critical understanding of the structures underlying and shaping the familiar world of daily experience. (p. 39, original emphasis)

By drawing attention to alternatives to what, for us, feels "natural and inevitable," this kind of speculation may allow new critical insights into the ideological structuring of our lives that we ignore because we were born into them. The presumption of a library that offers windows and doors to moments in the past works both as a simple plot device and a critical re-presentation of what we mean by a library.[6]

Comics, television, and fiction writer Warren Ellis (2009) describes this critical aspect when discussing what he calls "the central problem" of science fiction, which

> stands in a speculative zone from which to consider aspects of the present condition.... It needs...a piece of the future, of novelty, of something as yet unseen.... Faced with a line like "the door dilated," the brain has to do a little extra work to make it make contextual sense.... you accept the experience of *processing strangeness and applying it to the world you know.* (p. 48, my emphasis)

In this estimation, the strangeness or difference provoked by speculative fiction and the work it makes us do may also reveal to us this very same condition—strangeness, a feeling of something foreign—in the present, everyday world. And the constant feeling of the foreign-ness of the present may be especially salient given the increasingly shortened cycles of technological innovation in which, in technologist Kevin Kelly's (2017) words, "We are morphing so fast that our ability to invent new

[6] More on libraries in the concluding chapter.

things outpaces the rate we can civilize them" and so "Endless Newbie is the new default for everyone, no matter your age or experience" (pp. 8, 13). This gap in living is what Warren Ellis (2015) calls our Science Fiction Condition. In words that seem to invoke Clarke's maxim, he claims:

> The central metaphor is magic. And perhaps magic seems an odd thing to bring up here, but magic and fiction are deeply entangled, and you are all now present at a séance for the future. We are summoning it into the present. It's here right now. It's in the room with us. We live in the future. We live in the Science Fiction Condition, where we can see under atoms and across the world and across the methane lakes of Titan. ("How to See the Future")

The difference between Arthur C. Clarke's technology-that-is-indistinguishable-from-magic and Ellis's summoning is that, in the former, encounter with advanced technology is a bewildering surprise. Ellis argues the other direction. His point is that we should recognize how impossible our world is *right now*. I am at once both a dupe scratching at my magical glass rectangle like the obelisk in Clarke's *2001* and a magician who uses it to conjure—or purchase through Amazon—whatever I want. That is, I need to recognize the ways in which the future has found a place at the center of my life. Steven Shaviro (2024) asserts, "If the past still lingers in the present, then futurity already haunts the present—even before it arrives and even if it never does" (p. 11). In an analog to the hauntological relation between the past and present that Derrida described, the future haunts me as that impossible foreign center around which (my) life organizes.

It has become commonplace by now to insist that science fiction isn't predictive, but is—in terms of Aristotle's rhetorical brands—*deliberative*. Science fiction is an argument about what we should want or should do. At least, it is a gesture at what is desirable. The usual example is the original *Star Trek* communicator, which didn't predict flip phones as much as inspire later mobile phone designers. Of course, we have gone way beyond that now, since "Captain Kirk had to tune his fucking communicator and it couldn't text or take a photo that he could stick a nice

Polaroid filter on" (Ellis, 2015, "How to See the Future"). At best, the argument made by the *Star Trek* communicator was that maybe, in the future, pocketable personal communication will be both useful and desirable. Science fiction as a prediction about what futures I could possibly have is always— either in the details or completely—wrong. As Shaviro (2024) argues: "To say that science fiction is about futurity is to say that envisions potentialities rather than actualities" and, since these are *potentials* that exist *right now*, "these futurities exist precisely *as* potentialities or anticipations" (p. 11). Potentialities and anticipations are useful grounds for arguments.

So, even if a book, movie, or television show makes an argument about where we might-or-should-be headed, it seems that it's also very much about where we are right now (in Aristotle's branding, it's *epideictic*). In her introduction to *The Left Hand of Darkness*, Ursula Le Guin (2019) claims that "Science fiction is not predictive; it is descriptive," then offers a novel in which many of the characters have no fixed genders, are "ambisexual" (p. xvi). The descriptive nature of the written science fiction that she's proposing shares with art generally and literature particularly an ambivalence or gap or contradiction, since "[t]he artist deals with what cannot be said in words.... The artist whose medium is fiction does this *in words*. The novelist says in words what cannot be said in words" (p. xx). To say something that can't be said is a hard thing. But if that thing can't be said, then maybe it can be talked *about*? *About* in the sense of moving around it, tracing its contours, so that we can see it in relief, as an absence that was already there that we didn't know about until it was contained.[7]

And the promise of this new container is that it can be filled up.

That promise is never met, though. It can't be. There is something that is impossible to *say*, to render into language or any other symbolic system in order to make sense of it, tame it. But this impossibility is precisely what makes writing, television, movies, and every other art possible. Because, if it can't be filled up, there is always room to keep trying. Failure is what keeps me going. Failure is what I *enjoy*, because

[7] *The shapes a bright container can contain*! per Roethke's "I Knew a Woman." More on this (kind of) in the next chapters.

failure opens me up to the possibility of getting something else. This is how desire functions as a cause.

You Can Only Ever Have Eaten Your Cake

Todd McGowan (2015) introduces the problematic nature of desire through cake. "An animal feels the instinct of hunger, and then it eats and finds satisfaction. We feel a desire for a piece of chocolate cake, but even as we're eating it, we think of what we might like to have later that would be better than the chocolate cake" (pp. 28–29). I take chocolate cake very seriously.

Imagine that I have a piece of chocolate cake for the very first time and it's amazing. No other chocolate cake afterwards can live up to that first—now gone—piece, even if most of the pieces of cake I eat from then on are empirically better. The vanishing (as I eat it) of that first piece of cake institutes a desire that didn't exist before and only exists now that the first piece is gone forever. I am haunted by that first piece of cake. And so I eat and eat to try to reclaim that first piece, and even master enough of baking to produce my own chocolate cakes. I have become a recognized expert on chocolate cakes. And I enjoy these cakes serially, as each failure to satisfy pushes me further into the varied and sometimes seedy world of chocolate cakes. But even the *best* chocolate cake is lacking insofar as it cannot stand up to the contingent, possibly mediocre first piece that, really, is nothing but a placeholder, since *any* piece of chocolate cake would have done the exact same job. Messing with Benjamin's authenticity a bit, it is the first to evoke the *aura* of the original while being simply one of many, many copies and variations. That initial piece of chocolate cake is at once special and inconsequential, authentic and an imitation, since it is both the beginning of an ongoing frustration and, at the same time, nothing distinctive at all.

The psychoanalytic truth is that this loss of the original-that-is-not-an-original figures a more fundamental, formal impossibility at the level of being that institutes desire as such. This mythic, wholly supposed *cause* of desire works as an object that is both the promise of satisfaction and, as Todd McGowan (2008) describes, "embodies the failure of any object of desire to satisfy the subject" (p. 71). No piece of cake—even one that is identical to the first one—will ever complete my quest. So, per Žižek (2001), as this mythic object "prevents the circle of pleasure from closing, it introduces an irreducible displeasure, but the psychic apparatus finds a sort of perverse pleasure *in this displeasure itself*, in the never-ending, repeated circulation around the unattainable, always missed object" (p. 48, original emphasis). This psychic apparatus is inescapable. The impossibility constitutes me as a subject of the unconscious and initializes a *failure* that I *enjoy*.

Knowingly and skillfully circulating around that impossibility, saying what cannot be said, is very much what Le Guin describes as the function of art.

To claim that there is something that can't be said is to claim that there is something that can't be represented (or re-presented). Freud called this primary repression, but it's important to quickly add that—like authenticity—this repression is primary only logically, not temporally. The repressed doesn't pre-exist repetition, but is instead generated *by* repetition. It's with the failure of the second piece of cake that things get rolling. But whether it's chocolate cake or something else, a formal distinction or difference is hailed by repeated (lack of full) enjoyment and is sustained and fed by that (dis)pleasure. Since, in the above example, *any* piece of chocolate cake could serve to set up desire, there isn't anything special about that first piece at all, *except* that it's first. Its lack of specialness is overwritten by a perception of loss at the first bite of a future piece of cake that sets desire in motion while also setting it up to always fail to find its object. The difference between the iterations of metonymy (here's one and here's one and here's one) and the iteration of repetition is precisely *difference*, here represented by (or narrativized as) failure. But repetition is not repeated failure. Alenka Zupančič (2008) argues as much:

> So the point is not that the constitutively missing (primarily repressed) signifier is the cause of repetition. Repetition is not the result of a failed representation, or the result of (primary) repression. It is not that the lack of the "right" signifier induces repetition (which would stop if the right

signifier were found again). Rather, repetition and primary repression are part of one and the same process. (p. 167)

The gap is introduced only once there are two. Repetition is therefore always also the repetition of the gap or impasse itself. *Authenticity* as discussed above is another way of figuring how the original is generated by the introduction of another,[8] but it is also a way of showing how the contingency of the first is then raised to the status of a primary, necessary, even mythic principle. However, the only way this temporal first instance can attain its mythic status is to be narrativized as something I've lost.

There are two issues to stress here. The first is that, given the failure of each iteration to fully account for or re-present that mythic lost object, what I begin to enjoy is repetition itself, and insofar as failure means more repetition, I enjoy my failure. I enjoy the failure of each new piece of cake I encounter as a difference from that original piece. I have no way of *knowing* the quality of that first piece outside of its differences from those that I encounter afterward: *that's not it and that's not it and that's not it*.... The promise is that, possibly, sometime in the future, I will have collected enough differences to reconstruct the pleasure of the mythic original by tracing its silhouette or connecting the dots. I will bake *about* it. Thus, the second issue is that moving from one to two (or, better, two to three) implies a sequence—a story or narrative or an idea of progress—as searching for the ultimate piece of chocolate cake points forward to an ultimate end to the search. The possibility of having a story depends on the second or third or ultimate already being there as a destination. And much like the virtual shelves in the great music archive from the previous chapter, a place in the bakery display case has been set aside for the final cake that is also a formal ideal.[9] So, narrative as such is always after the fact and is a way of trying to cover over the contingent relationship of the one and the others. If repetition is a mark of failure, narrative is the fantasy that hides that failure.

---

[8] More on this in the sixth chapter, in terms of both food and "life-like" dolls.

[9] See the section on Cause in the first chapter of my book *Contingency, Immanence, and the Subject of Rhetoric* (Richardson, 2013, pp. 27–33) for more on Aristotle's four causes and Kenneth Burke's reimagining of them.

This narrativization is always at work. These are the stories we tell about the world and about ourselves. The ego is nothing but a narrativizing of Jacques Lacan's famous split subject—a contingent subject that is not identical with itself, a subject that is constituted by the gap—as a coherent and recognizable "self" that is more or less autonomous.[10] But repetition is the insistence of the lie these stories are: the lie that is fantasy. Again, Zupančič (2008):

> repetition exists because there is no linear genesis of the subject (or, to put it the other way around: because there is a subject—the latter being precisely the effect of a dysfunction in the purely linear causality). The genesis of a subject always and necessarily involves a leap, and repetition at its fundamental is repetitious jumping, going back and forth between the edges of this leap. On this particular level repetition is clearly opposed to fantasy, which consists in filling in the gap in question, and transforming the constitutive leap into a linear story. Also, at its most fundamental, fantasy is fantasy about the origins (of the subject). (p. 169)

In this way, fantasy is primarily about failure turned into success, since it's a story proposing (impossible) satisfaction and the return of what never actually existed. Fantasy is never about satisfaction, but its infinite deferment. There is nothing worse, says Žižek, than having your fantasies actualized.[11] And while both Zupančič and Žižek are talking about the psychoanalytic kind of fantasy, the genre kind maps nicely to this economy, too. So many genre books are parts of continuing series for this reason. Frustration is the engine of desire.

Which is perhaps sometimes a good thing. If my desire for chocolate cake could ever be satiated completely, there would be no more reason to eat cake. Or—if we're talking about things other than cake—to get out of bed in the morning. Lack can be generative. As Mari Ruti (2017)

[10] Some people are uncomfortable with the definition of a subject as that which coalesces around a gap, but the fact of the gap is what allows change in the subject, since the subject is never discrete or autonomous.

[11] Responding to the awful "male-chauvinist platitudes about how, in being raped, women only get what they secretly wanted," Žižek (1997) writes, "To this commonplace, one should answer that (some) women may actually daydream about being raped, but this fact not only in no way legitimizes actual rape—it makes it even more violent" (p. 188).

explains, "the lack of complete satisfaction does not mean that there is no satisfaction to be had. If anything, the intrinsic impossibility of complete satisfaction is what sustains us as creatures of becoming and what allows us, over and again, to take up the inexhaustible process of producing meaning, including the process of signifying beauty" (p. 127).[12] The point to be had here, though, is that we enjoy failure or, to be more affirmational, we enjoy the (infinite) deferment of success. Failure is what allows me to say that I love chocolate cake and to ask for another piece.

And we can see how the deferment of satisfaction is perhaps the driving force behind not just bakeries, but capitalism more generally. Todd McGowan (2016) makes this point explicitly:

> The fundamental gesture of capitalism is the promise, and the promise functions as the basis for capitalist ideology. One invests money with the promise of future returns; one starts a job with the promise of a higher salary; one takes a cruise with the promise of untold pleasure in the tropics; one buys the newest piece of electronics with the promise of easier access to what one wants. In every case the future embodies a type of satisfaction foreclosed to the present and dependent on one's investment in the capitalist system. The promise ensures a sense of dissatisfaction with the present in relation to the future. (p. 11)

The promise of the future is the promise that what needs taking care of now will have been taken care of then. Whatever I lost will either be found or replaced with something even better. This is the belief grounding the economy of collectors' toys and comic book speculation, but such a nostalgia play is limited in scope. In fact, nostalgia for a simpler time in which I wasn't (consciously) aware of my entanglement in the discourse of capitalism, when toys just showed up (or didn't), is an example of capitalism's ability to assume even negative reactions to itself.

More often, though, instead of a nameable loss that needs addressing, what I feel most is a dissatisfaction with the present. Whatever I have now is clearly lacking the thing that makes it complete. But it is also clearly a step forward, toward having that thing in the future. If not with

[12] Lack as the engine of a non-capitalist engine for engagement is the best outcome, and is the subject of the concluding chapter.

the next iteration, then maybe with the one after that. In every case, my next whatever will be a better whatever. The engine of capitalism is belief in the better future.[13] A Future with Retsyn.

The trick is something like nostalgia in reverse. Instead of the (ill-defined and misremembered) best being behind me, it's up ahead, in the new job or restaurant or partner or television or the new, better smart phone. The capitalist future depends on projecting a better version of now that is at once just out of reach and is settled, waiting for me, since I know what (or at least *that*) I want and the customer is always right. There is a place prepared for that thing, and for me having it.

In what seems like a reversal of the chocolate cake phenomenon, Italo Svevo's 1923 novel *Zeno's Conscience* follows a protagonist named Zeno Cosini who, instead of looking to recapture some lost original enjoyment, is always looking to have his final cigarette. Each chapter ends with him smoking his "last" one. The joke, of course, is that the metonymy of identical cigarettes (here's one and here's one and here's one) denies the specialness of any particular instance. The lesson is that Zeno can never *have* his final cigarette, but only *have had* it. That this is the forward-facing version of the same operation is apparent insofar as we can never capture either the (mythical) original or the (equally mythical) final, but can only miss it.

In his elaboration of what Lacan called the discourse of capitalism, Stijn Vanheule (2016) makes exactly this point: "Capitalist discourse actively cultivates the semblance of dissatisfaction, as well as a fantasy of self-sufficiency, completeness and vitality" (p. 7). The dissatisfaction promoted by capitalism is of the not-yet variety, wherein each engagement (each purchase or investment of whatever sort) comes with a necessary acknowledgment that this doesn't quite do it for me but that it could, that it will.

Deferment is what makes consumer capitalism work for me in place of other relationships, as its constant circulation resembles activity on my part, only with very little exertion. Lacan's capitalist discourse is a radical modification of his prior four discourses: master, university, hysteric, and analytic. As Colette Soler (2014) explains:

[13] Capitalist belief is mirrored by the belief that defines masculinity in the next chapter.

> Each discourse—what Freud called civilisation—constructs a type of social bond, a sort of standard couple: master and slave, teacher and student, hysteric and master, and then psychoanalyst and psychoanalysand.... But there is no such possibility in the scientificised capitalist discourse. It is not a variant of the discourse of the master, and can only constitute a single, barely social bond between the individual and products. Indifferent as it is to "the business of love", it moves towards an increasing fragmentation and instability of social bonds, and leaves individuals always more exposed to insecurity and loneliness. (p. 191)

Each of the four prior discourses (Fig. 3.1) depends on an unconscious or repressed truth that supports those relationships but is never directly accessed or acknowledged. Instead, it is the site of knowledge, of what can't be written, but what guarantees at least a minimal distance by which a relationship with an other can be sustained.

This inaccessible support for the social bond guarantees that whatever message is sent to an other is always never complete or completely understandable. My first piece of chocolate cake wasn't the same as your first piece. Given this, our chocolate cake club is complicated by a fundamental misunderstanding of goals, but ignoring that misunderstanding is the foundation of our social contract and allows us to hold and enjoy our frequent meetings as failures.

The discourse of capitalism subverts that unconscious or repressed truth-support. For instance, in the master's discourse (Fig. 3.2), the unconscious (and therefore unacknowledged) support for the master is the split subject, the fact of the gap or impasse or impossibility. Ignoring that gap (repression) is what allows the master to take up the position of representative of an established and necessary order (this can be traced back to Aristotle's Mover, but also to the God by whom a

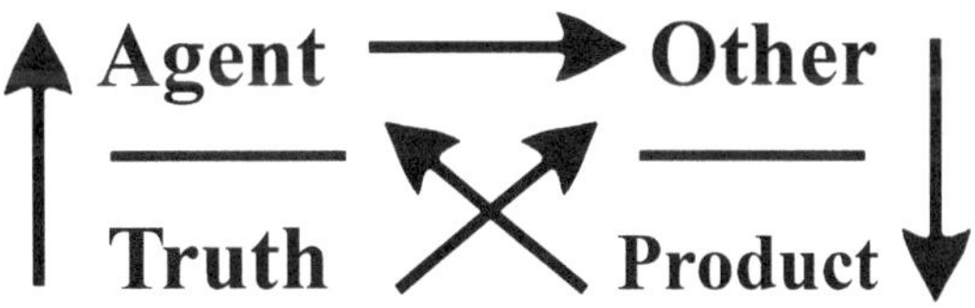

Fig. 3.1 The structure of discourse

monarch receives his divine right). The radical shift that Lacan describes as the capitalist discourse (Fig. 3.3) is one in which a split, lacking, castrated subject doesn't address an other directly. Instead, what in the prior discourses would be the unconscious truth supporting the subject's relationship with an other is here opened up in the form of a signifier, a product, through which I may access the other that has become what John Holland (2016) calls a "catalogue of satisfactions" (p. 114).

The effects of this new availability are double. First, it insists that my social bond with an other (the move from Agent to Other in the pre-capitalist mathemes) is now only possible via an intermediary object, a product or service that will always focus that rapport in commercial ways. Instead of the misunderstanding that founds a relationship and allows room for fantasy to take hold, this new discourse focusses any exchange through the lens of a product, service, or capital itself.[14]

And this is the second effect. Once the impasse or impossibility that complicates and slows the social relationship is elided in favor of an easy access via a stable, market-friendly key, finding a gap or crack through

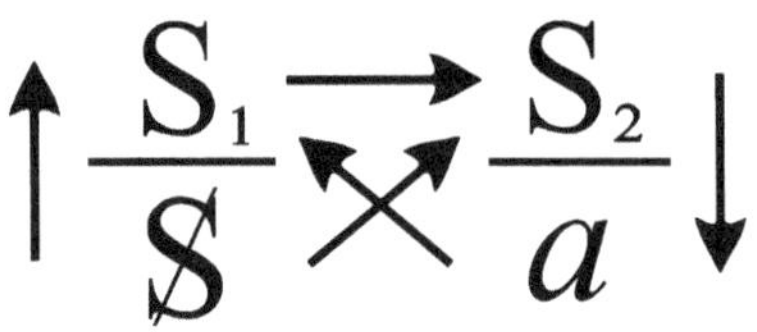

Fig. 3.2 The Discourse of the Master

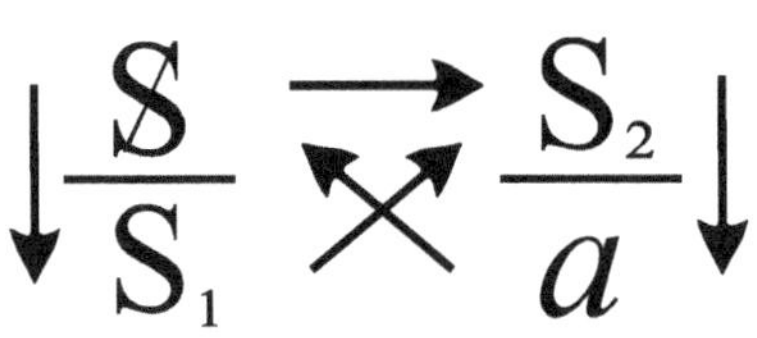

Fig. 3.3 The Discourse of Capitalism

[14] Running something—a government or school, for instance—like it is a business is precisely the narrowing of the possibilities of social bonds to one relationship via a surrogate that flattens difference and can therefore perpetuate itself across borders.

which to intervene—politically, economically, or psychoanalytically—becomes very, very difficult. The success of the capitalist discourse is that it doesn't stop writing itself. As Holland (2016) describes:

> It reproduces, in the field of the psychic and the social bond, the limitless movement that characterizes capital; both domains are dominated by the same sort of infernal machine. Once the circuit has been traversed and one returns to the beginning at [the split subject], nothing favors one's escape from this discourse and everything leads one, instead, to repeat the same path that has only just been taken. (p. 110)

The promise of the discourse of capitalism is that, in its constant circulation, there is no impasse, no way to acknowledge and traverse the fantasy,[15] no rupture in which I can potentially witness its failure or lack of permanence. Instead, the discourse accounts for discontent within the capitalist system by pushing the final answer perpetually further down the road. Again, Vanheule (2016):

> Within the capitalistic logic, the lack at the heart of subjectivity is not seen as a structural consequence of using signifiers, but an accidental frustration that can be remedied within the market of supply and demand….
> As a result, capitalist discourse implies a particularization of desire, treated as if it is a demand. Whereas in classic [Lacanian] discourse desire is singular in that it cannot be solved by means of the signifier, the capitalist discourse suggests that particular solutions for dealing with subjective division actually exist: the market is there to satisfy customers' demands. Consequently, at the point of desire, the capitalistic logic leads to exploitation: "the exploitation of desire, this is the big invention of capitalist discourse." (p. 7, his translation)

As a subject of capitalism, to the gap about which I coalesce (formal desire per Zupančič) is introduced a master signifier (a product, whatever) that grants access to the field of signifiers (products, commodities)

---

[15] More on traversing the fundamental fantasy in the concluding chapter.

that stands for the market as such. Through this master or first signifier—say, a new television or smart phone, but also an account on a social media service—my relationship to the market (Amazon, Walmart, Instagram, or whatever other "catalogue of satisfactions") is established and I have full access to all that the market can offer.

But that market is also evidence that there are more televisions and smart phones and, well, everything else that's available or just out of stock and, as a vast site of possibility, the marketplace demonstrates to me both the failure of this new particular television to meet every foreseeable need and—regardless of variations, or because of them—the impossibility of any of its contemporaries to completely satisfy, too.[16] Why so many options unless none of them are perfect? One answer may be that each consumer is different and has different needs and desires. And this would make sense if every product were bespoke, manufactured to meet the needs of a specific individual at a specific moment. But that's generally not the case, and so the catalogue of satisfactions also works to define my desires through pre-given options while at the same time allows me to believe that I'm special, that the choice is mine.[17]

The failure of the market to immediately satiate is, through the constant movement that capitalism enforces, converted into the promise of a future satisfaction only (ultimately) available through participation within the iterative cycle (this television is good enough right now, but barely), thereby translating my desire (which is by definition unsatisfiable) into a demand of and for the future and engendering a subject who can do nothing else but give itself to the cycle, since these are now the only terms available to me once I've bought in.

And as products have given way to subscription services, the cycling becomes explicit with the automatic payments from my checking account each month, an iteration of the same old service that nonetheless promises a new delight that will be available forever in the place prepared for it.

[16] The proliferation of social media influencing marks both a variety of ways to "live well" and a narrowing of performances of "the good life" to what can be consumed quickly.

[17] The previous chapter discussed this as mall-store rebellion.

If repetition is the engine of desire, then the engine of capitalism replaces repetition (and desire) with iterative cycles of supply and demand that project the promise of satisfaction into the future, narrativizing the formal impasse as a *not-yet* or *not-quite* or *to-come* such that every failure of every product is also a promise about a future that is already assumed with, in, and by the present. Here, iterative production cycles take the place of singular repetition and demand for the new replaces desire for what I feel has been lost. The irony is that, once the system is set in motion, instead of feeling caught in capitalist iterative circulation, movement in this system *seems to be* spurred *by me*. Samo Tomšič (2015) argues "This structural tendency generates the fetishist appearance of self-engendering value, which causes the 'desire for participation' in the presupposed essence of wealth" (p. 162). As I am supplied by the system with new iterations of products or wealth abstraction opportunities, my demand for the new, for progress and growth, is both a result of the discourse I've been injected into and a sign of my investment in it. Tomšič continues to explain that "In order for this obscenity of capitalism to be socially implemented with success, it must be accompanied by an ideological fiction" of growth and health regardless of the political or economic facts (p. 162). Belief in the sanctity of market forces necessitates any failure to be registered as a personal failure and not as a systemic problem.

The supply-and-demand product version of iteration-as-narrative we all know well is easily illustrated in the refresh cycles of tech hardware. As an Endless Newbie, a new iteration of my phone each year guarantees that I am on the right track, that each *better* is a step along the track toward the *best* (this is also where we find religious "fan-boy" arguments about innovation: Google or Microsoft invents and Apple perfects, etc.). But the truth is that there isn't a vacant shelf in the future being held for the phone that finally does it all *for me*, in part because the "all" keeps changing as circumstances change. And (as much as the fantasy of a stable subject—the fundamental fantasy—works to hide it) so does the "me."

The linear story of technological progress up to now is a fantasy narrative. And whatever problems are being addressed by new phones (or televisions or jobs or restaurants or partners) are already old problems, as the new phone opens up new possibilities that it can't help but just fail to realize. These new potentials are either immediately subsumed within the constant circulation of the discourse of capitalism as a new cause for investment (market disruption is thus already part of the market), or (with more hope) they remain hidden potentials that are exploitable gaps in the smooth running of the machinery.[18]

Steven Shaviro (2015) makes this latter point about potential in technology:

> There is no preexisting "possibility space" for any medium—or, more generally, for any technology. The development and deployment of a technology generates its own affordances and constraints, which themselves may differ under different economic and social conditions. Technological development will always have a speculative (and nonutilitarian) dimension. (p. 17–18)

Technology—even caught within the circulation of capital—doesn't *necessarily* advance some grand upward trajectory in a fantasy of growth.[19] Instead of iteration, it may be possible to recognize, even within such a totalizing system, the kind of rupturing repetitions that generate their own affordances, which may in turn allow me to break (from) the constant circulation. While impossibility as such is formal and necessary, the instances in which I encounter that impasse are always partial, specific, contingent, and *right now*. They are not located in the future or the past, but are recognizably disturbances of or in the narrative of perfectibility upon which both nostalgia and capitalism depend.

Future's Past

Cyberpunk as a subgenre of science fiction certainly found its legs by the early 1980s, and the aesthetics of cyberpunk originally demonstrated its politics. William Gibson's famous dictum from 1981's *Burning*

---

[18] The sixth chapter takes up a broad understanding of hacking as a mode of exploiting gaps.

[19] Or fantasies of escape, as with some billionaires' projects to colonize Mars. Masculine escape is discussed in the fifth chapter.

Chrome that "the street finds its own use for things" indicates a future in which old, discarded technology—replaced to maintain the iterations of consumer capitalism—is repurposed for subsistence and resistance by a disenfranchised population. In film, the remains of the past in the present of this future are illustrated by typewriters tied to view screens in *Blade Runner* (1982) and the vast networks of pneumatic tubes shuffling paperwork in *Brazil* (1985). These antiques pushed into the future refuse the romantic and welcoming skeuomorphism of "folders" on the desktops of home and office computers from the 1980s onward. Instead, they insist on the clumsiness of bureaucracy beyond any technological innovation (and, especially in the case of *Brazil*, bureaucracy is one of those technologies). Of course, cyberpunk as an aesthetic survived beyond the 1980s and it became difficult to imagine a future that was otherwise. We were stuck with the same dark future for decades, as it lost its revolutionary appeal to fashion (*The Matrix*, 1999) and nostalgia. To be fair, though (as discussed in the fifth chapter), *Blade Runner* as a *noir* film set in the future was already a nostalgic project, bridging the past of popular fiction and the future of corporate overreach that we now find ourselves enjoying.

By projecting fulfillment into the past or the future, nostalgia and capitalism narrativize the gap or impasse, thus treating the impasse as a deficit that will have been overwritten instead of the foundational impossibility of completeness. Both try to cover the gap described earlier as ambivalence and contradiction with projections away from the present, so that the present is always *about* some other, more perfect time.[20] Both are ways of enjoying the present impasse by narrativizing either as

[20] Looking to the next chapter, lack, and its narration as loss, only exist at the introduction of the signifier that initially functions to distance the subject from the other (we can read this developmentally or formally). Once the signifier becomes stabilized with and by the network (the Symbolic Order), distance from its neighbor (and the structures that support that distance) becomes reified as "Law." The phallic signifier—as a signifier without a signified—is thus a product of the networks function of fixity. As the signifier for Law, the phallic signifier is only ever a mark of the lack, loss, or distance endemic to the symbolic, while at the same promising that lack/loss/distance is "natural" and not contingent.

fantasy (the Past) or through the upgrade cycles of promise (the Future of capitalism).[21]

Some speculative fiction exploits this coincidence of impossibility and the present. That is, as Steven Shaviro (2015) puts it: "science fiction is not about the actual future but about the futurity that haunts the present" (p. 2). The futurity he posits is perhaps what William Gibson had in mind in his famous "the future is already here—it's just not very evenly distributed" and is precisely what Warren Ellis calls the Science Fiction Condition (Knapp, 2013). That Gibson's aphorism, Shaviro's futurity, and Ellis's Condition all insist on the *presence* of The Future indicates that the future is the perpetual *potential* of the present. Instead of convincing us of the consistency of the world (the job of fantasy world-building) or treating the present as rehearsal for the future (capitalism), this kind of speculation would instead demonstrate the impossible as kind of immanence, an aporia that resists easy assimilation and instead indicates that things now can be otherwise.

In a different idiom, we could say that this is the rhetorical dimension of the Science Fiction Condition. The potential might be what Diane Davis (2010) calls rhetoricity, "an affecta*bility* or persuad*ability*—that is the condition for symbolic action" (p. 2, original emphasis). Like Ellis's Condition, rhetoricity would be interior to the present but foreign, unhomely—what Lacan and Jacques-Alain Miller calls extimacy—and is what allows for any deployment of persuasion or affect. And, certainly, speculative work is all about persuasion and affect.

As a kind of aside, we might ask, what does it mean to say that it is a condition, sci-fi or otherwise?

- "Condition" can mean *circumstance*, which jibes with the contingency discussed above, since the circumstances in which I find myself are contingent upon a number of known and unknown elements.
- In a related sense, condition can also mean *constraint*, most obviously illustrated in the if/then relationship. This implies contingency, too, I suppose, since the constraints can change or vary in degree.

[21] In contrast, per Le Guin, art often reveals that distance between what we actually have and the impossibility that sustains desire, and then refuses to cover that gap over. Art is about what can't be said but can be talked about.

- But condition can also simply mean the state of something which, having to do with the overall condition, doesn't feel very contingent. That something is in good or bad condition means that it is maybe closer to an objective or formal state than a contingent one.

Conditions have very much to do with the present and can be the cause for all sorts of behavior. The condition of my house's roof after a Texas hailstorm is maybe a good example of how condition as circumstance works as what Aristotle would have called an *efficient* cause. Ice balls break shingles, roofers invade to help assess damage, and insurance agents are deployed. This is all contingent upon the location of my house and the age of my roof and probably a lot of other elements I can't keep track of.

These contingencies depend upon relationships like geography and weather, of course, but also on *material* properties like the kind of shingles the roof has and hail being made of ice and ice being hard. Conditions as circumstances are closely related to material properties, but this should in no way undercut the contingency of those circumstances.

Materiality isn't formal or final (just as biology is not destiny). Ice can melt, etc. But the materiality of contingent conditions is maybe a good way to get at another, related understanding of condition: that of constraint. These are the types of conditions under which this kind of roof damage occurs. The most obvious use of constraint is the if/then relationship: if hail strikes my roof with sufficient force in its weakest spots, then the roof is compromised.

But condition can also mean the state of something, and this is where it comes closest to the *formal*. My roof may not have suffered any damage and, at least right now, it can be classified by an objective, insurance-friendly Good. The difficulty here is that the assessment of my roof is really a comparison, and not a very close one. There may be objective criteria by which every roof marked Good is measured, but these criteria do not (and cannot) account for all of the differences among the multitude of roofs. The assessment of a particular roof does not arise "organically" from the particulars of the roof in question but is, by necessity, an evaluation pushed upon the roof from the outside. The criteria were established long before the insurance agent encounters the roof. The agent's job is to account for how my roof more or less conforms.

So, insurance may at first seem an example of (the most boring kind of) speculative fiction, insofar as insurance is a literal investment in the future being very much like the present. But by externalizing and generalizing the Good, it does much the same work as nostalgia and capitalism. Except instead of projecting the better into the past or future, insurance lowers the bar of the formal Good to a comforting Good Enough by ignoring the specific, material differences that might inspire architects or writers.

That is, instead of opening up to contingency, to the gap or inconsistency or impossibility that hides inside the everyday, insurance bets that life is more of the same and invests in transcribing time itself into actuarial tables, expenses, and payouts.

In any case, the assertion that rhetoricity as extimacy is a condition for persuasion and affect jibes pretty well with a general definition of the rhetorical I proposed elsewhere: "Rhetoric as a practice may be that which addresses the contingent, foreign element internal to the subject" (2013, p. 18), especially if we imagine the "condition" as one version of the gap described above. Any rhetorical act would then be a recognition of fantasy-work as just that, and would look to exploit the impasse or gap that fantasy tries to cover over.

We can also recognize the rhetoricity of technology in technology's "speculative dimension," and any rhetorical act would then be an exploitation of those new affordances and constraints. It is here, in this treatment of technology, that we find science fiction that resists the easy reconciliations of the fantasy- or capitalist-inflected kind. This is true even in those versions in which capitalism and fantasy intersect to offer (sexual) products.

Bibliography

Benjamin, W. (1969). *Illuminations: Essays and reflections* (H. Arendt, Ed. & H. Zohn, Trans.). Schocken Books.

Bould, M. (2002). The dreadful credibility of absurd things: A tendency in fantasy theory. *Historical Materialism, 10*(4), 51–88.

Burke, K. (1969b). *A Rhetoric of Motives.* University of California Press.

Clarke, A. C. (1968). Clarke's third law on UFO's. *Science, 159*(3812), 255–255.

Davis, D. (2010). *Inessential solidarity: Rhetoric and foreigner relations.* University of Pittsburgh Press.

Ellis, W. (2009). *Shivering sands* (First Edition edition). International Electrophonic Unit.

Ellis, W. (with Strunk, R.). (2015). *Cunning plans: Talks by Warren Ellis* (E. Zitron, Ed.). SUMMON Books.

Fawaz, R. (2011). "Where No X-Man Has Gone Before!" mutant superheroes and the cultural politics of popular fantasy in postwar America. *American Literature, 83*(2), 355–388.

Guin, U. K. L. (2019). *The left hand of darkness: 50th anniversary edition.* Ace Books.

Hall, D. (2004). Civil war reenactors and the postmodern sense of history. *Journal of American Culture, 17*, 7–11.

Hall, G. (2015). Selective authenticity: Civil war reenactors and credible reenactments. *Journal of Historical Sociology, 29*(3), 413–436.

Haraway, D. J. (2016). *Staying with the trouble: Making kin in the chthulucene.* Duke University Press.

Holland, J. (2016). The capitalist uncanny. *S: Journal of the Circle for Lacanian Ideology Critique*, *8*(0). http://www.lineofbeauty.org/index.php/S/article/view/60

Kelly, K. (2017). *The inevitable: Understanding the 12 technological forces that will shape our future (reprint edition).* Penguin Books.

Knapp, A. (2013, August 1). *Warren ellis talks about his new novella and living in a science fiction present*. Forbes. https://www.forbes.com/sites/alexknapp/2013/08/01/warren-ellis-talks-about-his-new-novella-and-living-in-a-science-fiction-present/

McGowan, T. (2007). *The real gaze: Film theory after lacan.* State University of New York Press.

McGowan, T. (2008). *The real gaze: Film theory after lacan.* State University of New York Press.

McGowan, T. (2015). *Psychoanalytic film theory and the rules of the game.* Bloomsbury Academic.

McGowan, T. (2016). *Capitalism and desire: The psychic cost of free markets.* Columbia University Press.

Miéville, C. (2009). Cognition as ideology: A dialectic of SF theory. In C. Miéville & M. Bould (Eds.), *Red planets: Marxism and science fiction* (pp. 231–248). Pluto Press.

Murfin, R. C., & Ray, S. M. (Eds.). (2008). *The bedford glossary of critical and literary terms* (3rd edition). Bedford/St. Martin's.

Richardson, T. (2013). *Contingency, immanence, and the subject of rhetoric*. Parlor Press.

Richardson, T. (2021). Home bodies: Prosthetic people and economies of desire. In C. Neill (Ed.), *Lacanian perspectives on blade runner 2049* (pp. 103–119). Springer International Publishing.

Ruti, M. (2017). *The ethics of opting out: Queer theory's defiant subjects*. Columbia University Press.

Shaviro, S. (2015). *No speed limit: Three essays on accelerationism*. Univ Of Minnesota Press.

Shaviro, S. (2024). *Fluid futures: Science fiction and potentiality*. Repeater.

Soler, C. (2014). *Lacan—The unconscious reinvented: The unconscious reinvented*. Routledge.

Tomšič, S. (2015). *The capitalist unconscious: Marx and Lacan*. Verso Books.

Vanheule, S. (2016). Capitalist discourse, subjectivity and lacanian psychoanalysis. *Frontiers in Psychology*, *7*. PubMed. https://doi.org/10.3389/fpsyg.2016.01948

Vint, S. (2014). *Science fiction: A guide for the perplexed* (annotated edition). Bloomsbury Academic.

Žižek, S. (1997). *The plague of fantasies (first edition)*. Verso.

Žižek, S. (2001). *Enjoy your symptom!: Jacques Lacan in hollywood and out (2 edition)*. Routledge.

Zupančič, A. (2008). *The odd one in: On comedy*. The MIT Press.

4

Home Bodies

The first season of the television show *Mad Men* (2007) takes place in 1960. I wasn't alive then and, even if I were, my people never, ever made it to Madison Avenue, or even New York City. It is as alien a world as any science fiction. What I *can* compare the impeccable staging of this series to are the movies and television programs I've seen that were actually made back then and, in that comparison, the staging of *Mad Men* is unimpeachable. Much more accomplished than the history-gestures of *Star Trek*, the ashtrays, suits, and glassware are authentically period appropriate. But this precision sets up an ambivalence. While it certainly looks like (what I know of) 1960 New York, what this twenty-first Century staging allows—the scenes of sex, overt racism, and emotional cruelty (or at least the relatively graphic way they are treated)—don't resemble anything that would have—or in most cases could have—been *shown* in 1960 (except, perhaps, comically). *Mad Men* is *really* twenty-first-century television. Somehow (like remastered old music), the series places us contemporary folks back then, generating at once a kind of

Some of the discussion of the television series began as a short article Richardson, T. (2010). The Looks of Men: Doubling and Nostalgia in Mad Men. *Popular Culture Review* 21(1), 21–31.

T. Richardson, *Nostalgia, Fantasy, and the Futures of Masculinity*, The Palgrave Lacan Series, https://doi.org/10.1007/978-3-032-23921-1_4

nostalgia for their "simpler" sexual and racial politics while also allowing the performance of blatant racism and sexism that generally wouldn't be okay in a twenty-first-century series (at least, without characters suffering consequences). And it does this without the kind of irony that would allow us to forgive the behavior as something we've outgrown. They are *like* us, but they aren't *us*.

The ambivalence is precisely the point. *Then*, overt racism and sexism were apparently *de rigueur*. *Now*, we can be more sexually explicit, more violent, more whatever. And on television, we can have our *then* now by placing our *now* back then. But the result of this swapping is more than just a fun combination of anachronisms, since we understand that sex of course *happened* back then, if only after somewhat passionate kissing and a slow fade to black. And, more troubling, the daily sexism and racism *then* is still with us. After all, *then* is the America that was, by at least some estimations, Great. The effect is a kind of warping, much like that of a Möbius strip, and this warp is where we find pleasure in programs like *Mad Men*. What we enjoy and what repulses us become confused as the past and present commingle in performance.[1]

As the previous chapters argue, our treatment of the past—and especially what we *enjoy* about the past which is supposedly missing now—may indicate what we want out of our fantasy of the future, too. A past recollected in tranquility can just as easily be a future, as long as the requisite distance is there. This chapter is about some of the forms that distance can take, especially in terms of masculinity à la Jacques Lacan's elaborations of sexuation. Discussions of enjoying the future come later in this chapter via the films *Her* (2014) and *Ex Machina* (2015), but it's worth spending a little time in the "past" of *Mad Men*, just to set the bearings.

[1] An obvious example with this move in a series set contemporarily would be *The Sopranos* (the shows share an executive producer), where we're dealing for the most part with an alien subgroup who don't live by the same rules we do (this portrayal is one reason Italian American anti-defamation groups were upset), so one way of *imagining* the people of the past would be as an ethnic and cultural minority.

The Clique of Man

Titled "Babylon," episode six of the first season of *Mad Men* is structured around two separate advertising accounts. One is for Israeli tourism and is the impetus for the protagonist Don Draper's examination of the "research" available to him, consisting primarily of head shots of beautiful Israeli models, photographs of concentration camp atrocities, and the novel *Exodus*. At the same time, the office has taken over a campaign for Belle Jolie lipsticks. The copywriters are at a loss as to how to proceed with the latter ("I don't speak moron") and so decide to "throw it to the chickens" (Weiner et al., 2007). All the secretaries in the office are brought into a room containing rows of tables and chairs, the door is (pointedly) locked behind them, and the women are asked to pick their favorites from a collection of lipsticks, try them, and then answer survey questions asked by a stern German woman. The trick is that all the men in the series, including their boss Roger, are hidden behind one-way glass in a room with a full bar and lounge chairs. That is, all the men except Don Draper. At various points, one of the men uses a marker to circle and X the faces of women who are obliviously using the other side of the glass as a mirror, another asks if anyone minds if he takes off his pants, and the lead secretary Joan (a bombshell redhead who knows what's going on) seems to look directly at them through the glass, turns her back to them, and then bends to lean over a table. The men stand and salute.

Here we have an exact performance of the classic male gaze described by Laura Mulvey in her influential 1975 essay, "Visual Pleasure and Narrative Cinema," where "The determining male gaze projects its fantasy onto the female figure, which is styled accordingly. In their traditional exhibitionist role women are simultaneously looked at and displayed, with their appearance coded for strong visual and erotic impact so that they can be said to connote *to-be-looked-at-ness*" (p. 11). This now-standard understanding of the male gaze posits that viewers identify with the male characters. However, the episode's almost perfect rendering of Mulvey's gaze also complicates that gaze via the introduction of the one-way glass, so that what our attention is drawn to—what makes this scene even more uncomfortable—isn't what and who the men are looking at, but *how* they are viewing, separated by a distance, hidden in a way that "beats the hell out of x-ray specs." Quickly, the one-way glass becomes a re-presentation of the television screen itself and, instead of enjoying the masculine specular fantasy Mulvey calls gaze, we're confronted with our own participation in such fantasies and must instead recognize therein our own desire to watch. Here, Mulvey's gaze is really Lacanian fantasy, and the gaze is to be found elsewhere.

In the introduction to *The Real Gaze: Film Theory After Lacan* (2008), Todd McGowan counters Mulvey's formulation by asserting: "The gaze is a blank point—a point that disrupts the flow and the sense of the experience—within the aesthetic structure of the film, and it is the point at which the spectator is obliquely included in the film.... As the indication of the spectator's dissolution, the gaze cannot offer the spectator anything resembling mastery" (p. 8). This gaze is, according to Lacan (1998), the object cause of desire (*objet a*) as it is rendered visible (p. 105). Thus, Slavjo Žižek (1997) makes much the same point as McGowan when discussing the "zero-level pornographic picture" as "that of a woman displaying her genitals *and* defiantly returning the gaze.... The camera's eye here is the object-cause which curves the space, the third intruder which 'spoils the game'..." so that "[t]he gaze is thus not where one would expect it...but in the traumatic object/hole which transfixes our look and concerns us most intensely—the model's eyes staring at us here are, rather, to remind us: 'You see, I'm watching you observing my gaze...'" (pp. 178, 179). As viewers, we are implicated. While Žižek's pornographic image isn't quite ready for prime time, Joan smiling through the glass and then bending over the table certainly performs a television-friendly approximation.

But this staging of masculine fantasy is actually two scenes interrupted by another in which Don Draper is meeting with Rachel, the owner of a 5th Avenue department store who is both the object of Draper's interest and Jewish. At this point, it's important to recall that a flashback to Draper's childhood at the beginning of the episode is there to remind us in part that Don Draper is also Dick Whitman and that he has escaped a depressing, abusive home on the farm by inventing his life through various lies. He is also the sole male character absent from the Belle Jolie lipstick-focus-group viewing party. This last is no accident.

Draper seems to be the 1960s masculine ideal. He's successful, charming, the one man who—at least to the other men in the office for whom he is a model—seems uncastrated. He is smarter than the other men; he drinks and works harder than the other men; he is (or seems to be) all-around better than the men of the office, including his boss, Roger. And he has his own women. Draper has a beautiful wife in the suburbs (Betty, who is perhaps the perfection of the secretaries in the room) and a bohemian New York City girlfriend, in addition to whatever Rachel is to become. He is presented as Freud's mythical primal father. That Draper is necessarily excluded from the sad spectator scene is not an accident of the plot.

From the standpoint of the other men in the series, we can see that Draper's absence sustains them *as a group* insofar as they are all linked together by an essential not-being-Don-ness. That is, the men of the office form a set—Men of the Office—which is completed by the exclusion of Draper. In the top left of his graphs of sexuation from *Seminar XX*, Lacan (1999) argues that the masculine set is determined by the uncastrated exception so that:

> $\exists X \overline{\phi X}$marks that there is one (Freud's Primal Father, or here the uncastrated Draper) who does not fall under the phallic function, who is not castrated, effectively allowing for the delimiting of the set of all men by positing the exception or necessarily excluded term, and
> $\forall X \phi X$indicates that therefore all men fall under the phallic function or, as Lacan puts it, "it is through the phallic function that man as whole acquires his inscription." (p. 79)

This uncastrated, primal father is mythic and, like the cake of the previous chapter, myth is a way of explaining away lack as loss.

What Lacan describes is the exception that proves the rule, the logic of which is clearly laid out in teen high school comedies in which often, early on, a tour of the various cliques is performed for the benefit of the audience via a surrogate character. *Heathers* (1989), *Clueless* (1995), and *Mean Girls* (2004) are my family's touchstones, but there are many other examples. The reason for the almost Aristotelian categorization and hierarchization so early in such films is to establish the boundaries that the main character (sometimes a new kid, someone without baggage) is likely to later cross. The listing of these cliques in *Mean Girls*—Art Freaks, Burnouts, Cheerleaders, Cool Asians, Desperate Wannabes, Freshmen, Girls Who Eat Their Feelings, Preps, ROTC Guys, Sexually Active Band Geeks, among others—is another way of saying that these are not members of the presiding group, that they are "not Plastics." In *Heathers*, the ruling group (three Heathers and a Veronica) visits each of the other groups in the school cafeteria under the excuse of a school poll. The power play, though, is to remind each of the other groups that Heathers ask and others answer. The power such a dominant group has access to is wholly a function of its ability to exclude and, as almost every one of these films performs, exclusion is a function of insecurity, a lack of certainty, the fact that there is no *positive* characteristic that binds the group together. No individual Plastic or Heather can live up to the ideal, and this failure (along with the anxiety it provokes) is the phallic function that defines the group. Fantasy is the promise that success, Plasticity, is possible.

In *Mad Men*, the phallic function is precisely castration as the mark or cut that is the fundamental lack or negativity around which the subject coalesces and it is what allows for the collection of all these (masculine) subjects under one heading, thereby allowing for the signifier *Man*. Important here is that *Mad Men* does not *assume* a masculine subject, but instead explicitly performs the fantasy under which masculinity (as *failure*) is established and maintained. These men perform *for other men* in order to signal that they belong.

"Individuals are Wonderful"

So, while the other men enjoy the secretaries, Don Draper is meeting Rachel for lunch. The problem he's there to discuss with her stems from the new advertising account for Israeli Tourism. Up to this point, the episode has obliquely conflated Jewishness with femininity in pretty troubling ways, so that (for instance) the printed material Don has gone through contains both photos of attractive Israeli models *mixed in* with black-and-white images of Holocaust victims. After a close shot of these stacked on Don's desk, the episode cuts to secretaries at the agency captured, locked into the room with the lipsticks and a German interrogator.

In the beginning of the scene with Rachel, Don explains that he's looking for advice about the Israeli tourism account, to which Rachel responds, "And I'm the only Jew you know in New York City?" Don replies, "You're my favorite" and, soon after, accidentally spills some of his drink. In the first of two intimate moments, Rachel uses her napkin to dab at his tie and, while looking into his eyes, mumbles, "You're usually so put together." (Of course, Don really is "put together," since his is an assumed identity.) As Don begins to ask questions, Rachel balks at being treated as an expert, at one point saying "I don't know what I can say. I'm American. I'm really not very Jewish. If my mother hadn't died having me, I could have been Marilyn instead of Rachel, no one would know the difference." Of course, she's referring explicitly about being Jewish, but given the confusion of the Jewish and the feminine in the episode up to this point, Draper's immediate response, "What *is* the difference," can't help but resonate at the level of sexuation, too.

Rachel explains that Jews have lived in exile for a long time and suggests that they have managed so well because "we thrive at doing business with people who hate us." Don responds, "I don't *hate* you." "No," says Rachel, "individuals are wonderful…" and Draper interrupts, "That's not what I meant." Rachel softens, and talks about how a country is important and, though she doesn't want to live there, "it just has to be. For me it's more of an idea than a place." Don then takes her hand across the table (the second intimacy) and says "Utopia." "Maybe," responds Rachel, who then removes her hand. She explains that "they taught us at Barnard" the two meanings the Greeks had for the word: "the good place" and "the place that cannot be." Abruptly, Rachel excuses herself and leaves.

It is clear that Rachel's Jewishness and femininity are connected, constructing her as an amplified Other, an other whom Draper doesn't hate, one who has the answers he needs both professionally (this is the excuse for the meeting) and privately. But she doesn't have those answers, except insofar as she introduces the fundamental situation of exile. Rachel's parsing of the word *utopia*—The Good Place and The Place That Can Never Be[2]—might be read in terms of fantasy and desire.

As fantasy, The Good Place may be a return to what has lost been lost—a homeland, sure, but also sexual rapport that *was* complete and perfect and is *now* missing but might be realized in the future. As we saw in the previous chapter, this is how fantasy works.

In "Babylon," along with the specular fantasy of the secretaries and the occasionally tender meeting between Don and Rachel, there are two other notable scenes between men and women. The first as Mother's Day is ending and Don and his wife Betty are going to bed. After some banter, they begin to kiss. Betty asks Don to turn off the light. He obliges, returns to bed, runs his hand up her thigh, and Betty says:

> "I want you so much. I thought about it all day."
> "Me, too."
> "No, I mean it. It's all I think about. Every day. I hear a car coming down the driveway; I put the kids to bed early, I make a grocery list, I make butterscotch pudding, I never let my hands idle; washing my hair; drinking my milk. It's all in a kind of fog because I can't stop thinking about this. I want you. So badly."
> "Shh. You have me; you do." (Weiner et al., 2007)

Of course, she doesn't have Don, at least not completely. Don is both an unfaithful husband and not really Don. But on its own, near the beginning of the episode, what appears is innocence and caring and, really, who wouldn't want that? Indeed, this is a domestic utopia in the first sense, a good place to be.

The scene between Don and Betty is directly mirrored later. Draper's boss Roger is having an affair with Joan, his secretary. Near the middle of the episode, we see them in a hotel room together, preparing to leave. Roger talks about wanting to get Joan her own apartment and Joan argues that she likes living with a roommate—Roger responds that he will get her a bird—and that she prefers the freedom that the status quo offers. Toward the end of the episode, we find Roger in the hotel room

[2] The impossibility is also a theme of *The Good Place* (2016) tv show, which offers various versions of "good" throughout its run.

waiting as Joan enters (apparently late). They talk and laugh and kiss, then Joan hears a noise and notices a covered bird cage on the table. Roger removes the cover and the bird tweets. For a moment, we see Joan's face from the other side of the cage, as if she is also behind bars. Roger says, "You can't blame a man for trying. I just hate the thought of having to share you" as he unzips her dress. Joan replies, "You don't have to share me now" as she pulls him down onto the bed, on top of her. "Mmm, Joanie, you smell good. I've been thinking about this all day." Joan asks Roger to cover the bird; he obliges, and returns to bed.

Clearly, the sexual roles have reversed here in interesting ways. Where we had the housewife Betty waiting around for her husband to come home, we now have a powerful and philandering husband who takes every opportunity to sneak away to be with his mistress. Where we had Don saying to his wife Betty "You have me; you do," we now have the more honest Joan protesting "You don't have to share me now." The difficulty is that this isn't a strictly one-to-one trade. The shot of Joan through the cage reminds us of the secretaries being locked in the room with lipsticks (in that scene, Joan does the locking). And Betty asking for the lights to be turned off mirrors Joan wanting the birdcage covered insofar as both are reactions against being seen. Again, both reference the scopic reminiscent of the secretaries behind the glass.

One way of reading Lacan's famous *il n'y a pas de rapport sexuel* is as an insistence that the masculine and feminine positions are not complementary, not binary, nor are they concomitant operations that allow for easy exchange. If the category Man depends upon an excluded, uncastrated primal father of some sort as the exception that proves the rule, the feminine category is defined by its non-exclusion:

> $\overline{\exists X \phi X}$marks that there is not one who does not fall under the phallic function, so that the set of all women is unbounded and contingent, and $\overline{\forall} X \phi X$indicates that therefore all women do not fall wholly under the phallic function, thus eliding the possibility of a totalizing signifier for woman.[3] (78–79)

[3] Lacan, *Encore: The Seminar of Jacques Lacan,* 79. It is in this way we should understand Lacan's proclamation that woman is not-whole; she is not wholly defined by the phallic signifier.

While the masculine side elucidates particular tensions that define masculinity as, primarily, failure, the so-called feminine category is not so closed. As Calum Neill (2020) reminds us:

> Where the first, left-hand side is "the side of man," when it comes to the second side, the side we would typically describe as woman's, he tells us that "[a]ny speaking being whatsoever [...] whether provided with the attributes of masculinity [...] or not, is allowed to inscribe itself in this part." So, we have two positions available. One entails the inscription of "man," the other the inscription of "woman"; and yet this latter side is open to all. (p. 9)

Lacan's claim that the signifier Woman doesn't exist (as we'll see in the films later in this chapter) indicates that the unbounded, non-exclusionary properties of "the feminine side" allow for a great deal more potential.

Functionally, by conflating the Jewish and the feminine, the "Babylon" episode elucidates the fantasy-dimension that forms the common ground for both racism and sexism. For men. On the feminine side, there are a few more options. A woman may be the phallus (Betty, the secretaries) or have it (Joan). Here we find The Good Place, a space of lounge chairs, nicely stocked bars, and expensive hotel rooms that have been lost to us today but for which there is still a vacant spot waiting. We like to watch. And this Good Place is *authentic* insofar as it fits nicely into the hole we've prepared for it: nostalgia for lost excesses, sacrificed jouissance projected into the past. The Good Place offers a fantasy of completeness that is bolstered by what Todd McGowan (2008) sees as the primary work of mainstream cinema. Such a cinema of fantasy "allows the subject to relate to the lost object as an object that is simply out of reach. In fantasy, a spatial or temporal barrier, rather than an onto-logical one, intervenes between the subject and the lost object" (p. 24). This barrier is the temporal distance necessary for fantasy to take on a nostalgic form. The show functions nostalgically as a recollection of an

---

Returning to the high school movies tangent for a moment, the best illustration is probably *Heathers* (1989), in which a Heather can also be Veronica.

earlier time when things were simpler, men were real men and women were beautiful and both knew their places in the world.

But the feminine may also indicate a lack in the Other (the Other qua "the locus in which everything that can be articulated on the basis of the signifier comes to be inscribed," Lacan, 1998, p. 81). The feminine may also be drawn in terms of a relationship to the (lack in the) Other—S(barred-A)—such that "she is doubled, that she is not whole, since she can also have a relation with ϕ" (p. 81). It is important to stress here that the feminine subject (of whatever biological sex) is "not whole" because she is not constrained by the closing of the set that delimits the masculine position, depending as it does (per Zupančič, 2000) on an exception as "that which sets off the mechanism of exclusion (or differentiation), thus creating a set of all that comes under a certain condition" (p. 285). There is no Father, Prime Mover, First Piece of Chocolate Cake, or whatever.

In *The Psychoanalysis of Artificial Intelligence* (2021), Isabel Millar describes the difference between masculine and feminine sexuation this way: "masculinity is, formally speaking, a limit to forms of enjoyment and femininity is an unlimited mode of enjoyment. Not because women are not subject to castration, but because the function of non-castration does not determine their enjoyment. What characterizes a strictly masculine enjoyment is a limitation to only the phallic mode" (p. 94). After insisting on the masculine and feminine here are not defined by anatomy or genetics, she goes on to clarify:

> Not only does femininity operate according to a different logic than masculinity, but in a sense masculinity formally speaking is subsumed within femininity. In other words, being on the right-hand side of the graph does not preclude one from experiencing masculine sexuation and phallic enjoyment, conversely however being on the left-hand side of the graph limits one to a purely phallic mode of enjoyment and bounded mode of enjoyment which operates according to the logic of exception. (pp. 95–96)

The logic of the exception limits the set of the masculine and sustains that set as a failure. The exception is always the mark of failure. The not-whole of the feminine is thus the fact that the feminine may participate in the masculine economy (the Plastics and Heathers above) but is also not wholly defined by it. For the feminine, there are other possibilities.[4] And these alternatives have a different relation to desire as they suggest that, as a Place That Can Never Be, what was lost not only cannot exist now, but never has existed except in the search for it, as a failure of and in the Other. From the feminine (and, in the episode, also Jewish) subject position, homelessness is the essential and existential state of things.

In the final scene, Don goes to a café with his bohemian girlfriend and one of her other boyfriends (Don is no longer exceptional). Here, they discuss the commercialization of art in terms that evoke thoughts of the commercialization of sex. Of course, Don *makes* commercials. Finally, in order to both pull the themes of the episode together and to indicate the ambivalences discussed here, two men take the stage to perform Psalm 137, from which the episode takes its name. Over this lament of Jewish exile, we are shown Draper framed within the bent arm of his bohemian girlfriend and surrounded (via montage) by the other women in the episode. Don is "subsumed within femininity." We see Betty putting lipstick on their daughter, like the secretaries before. We see Rachel arranging men's ties at her store. And, finally, we see Joan and Roger leaving the hotel discreetly, separately, and ultimately waiting in silence at the curb, as far apart as the screen allows. Joan is carrying the bird cage.

By placing Draper amid the women, these visuals—along with the psalm of exile—precisely indicate Draper's doubling. On the one hand, he is (for the other men, at least) the enjoying primal father who functions as the exceptional, phallic support for the masculine fantasy that direct enjoyment (jouissance) is possible.[5] On the other hand, Draper stands for the not-whole. He is a stranger even to himself, and when he asked Rachel "What *is* the difference" between Jews and non-Jews,

[4] Alenka Zupančič (2018) backs up this explanation: "In truth, we are dealing with two different types of totality or 'whole', the difference conceptualized by Lacan as that between the 'all' and the 'not-all'. Crucial in understanding this difference is precisely to avoid the idea that "not-all" is the opposite of all, and thus of totality. Rather, the 'not-all' is 'all' to which something more gets added, it is "all" plus the point of view from which this all appears as 'all'" (p. 28).

[5] Or (for us viewers), that such enjoyment was possible way back when. The fact that we have effectively sacrificed that jouissance we presumably had access to in our past is paradoxically what allows us to enjoy the show.

between women and men, we have to recognize that Draper is also asking about himself and Dick Whitman, himself and the other men, etc., and that the only answer is exile. Something is not accounted for in the symbolic order. And that something is desire. If Don Draper can ever be considered at all ethical—and he only very occasionally can be—he is ethical insofar as he does not give up on his desire as such in order to settle for (and give in to) the failure and repetition that is simple masculine fantasy. Don doesn't settle. He is likewise excluded as both a mythic father (thus, from the scene behind glass) and as a (feminine) subject interrogating his place with/in the Other.

That so many of the rank-and-file characters of the series—gay or straight, male or female—are recognizably sexuated masculine serves to perform the everyday fantasies that keep many of us treading water (and, per the previous chapter, buying things). These characters also amplify those few characters who seem to offer more complicated possibilities: Don Draper in this episode, and also his new secretary Peggy (who doesn't want to be "another color in a box" in response to the lipsticks; Peggy's importance grows later in the series such that the show becomes every bit as much about her as it is about Don). But these exceptions, too, indicate fantastic solutions to an impasse that is formative and irresolvable. They promise that there exists (or at least existed) a way out of the repetition of failure.

Television series can give us very specific ways out through complicated fantasies that show the growth and change of characters over time because, ratings willing, a television series may have a very long time to work at it. Even in programs that are episodic, in which each episode is complete to itself, the variety of situations the writers invent to keep the show going also necessarily deepen our understanding of its characters. And, even for episodic programs but especially for those that develop story lines across episodes, the delay of any resolution enforces a sense of direction, of a journey toward a resolution of the desire each character stands for. When the conclusion of a series feels unsatisfactory to most people, it's likely because the audience has enjoyed the delay and repetitions so much that *any* resolution is going to feel weak by comparison. The failure to arrive is what we enjoy. Such is the jouissance of television.

Films, though, are sometimes different.

Movie Love

Since they tend to wrap up comparatively quickly, Hollywood movies often end more resolutely.[6] If modern television series promise a delayed, impossible resolution to the repetitions (and failures) we enjoy, Hollywood movies are *about* fantasy. I've argued in the previous chapter and elsewhere[7] that narrative storytelling often does the job of transmuting formative lack or impasse into feelings of loss and then offers up a resolution. A lack is something that never was. The promise of what's *lost* is that, eventually, it can be recovered.

Much of cinema takes up the most obvious lack or impasse for those of us here and now, the lack of sexual rapport, and tries to reconcile it for us. As McGowan (2011) argues:

> The romantic union has [its] ideological weight because it offers a fantasmatic solution to a fundamental social antagonism—that of sexual difference. The heterosexual romantic union that concludes so many films implies that antagonism can be surmounted, that a complementary relationship can be achieved.
>
> ....
>
> Throughout its history, the cinema—especially Hollywood cinema—has dedicated itself to the perpetuation of this idea more than any other task. By creating the romantic union, cinema assures us that antagonism is empirical rather than ontological and that we can always overcome it. (p. 84)

The promise is that sexual rapport is something we've lost, not something that's impossible. And movies can model the fantasy of what has been lost, making that fantasy seem available, if only eventually.

The word *eventually* is key. As television makes obvious, fulfillment must be deferred in order for us to enjoy the failure (of cake, of phone, of sex). Todd McGowan (2011) explains: "When we desire, we look to

---

[6] One of the difficulties with the Marvel Cinematic Universe (MCU) and other expansive franchises is that we're realizing that, instead of stand-alone cinematic experiences, these are actually big-budget tv episodes without resolution, since each has to set up the next and work in the "world."

[7] See Richardson, T. (2013). *Contingency, Immanence, and the Subject of Rhetoric*. Parlor Press.

the future as the time in which we will obtain the object and fulfill our desire," (pp. 12–13). McGowan isn't here talking explicitly about science fiction, but he could be.

As described in the previous chapter, "these futurities exist precisely *as* potentialities or anticipations" (Shaviro, 2024, p. 11) As potential, the future is always not yet, just beyond the horizon, a goal we only speculate about. And this speculation is almost literally *about* the future, moving around it, tracing its contours as we circle the object while always missing it. We just keep going. As Todd McGowan (2011) claims, "The only possibility that the future offers is that of a new form of repetition" (p. 12). And each repetition is a failure we enjoy.

And so we talk and write and make movies and tv that evoke this presence. Where the post-apocalyptic subgenre of the science fiction future may tend to find its support from primarily masculine fantasy (as mentioned in the previous chapter; the next chapter explores more), some films offer a futurity closer to home. Films like Spike Jonze's *Her* (2013) and Alex Garland's *Ex Machina* (2014) screen comfortable futures in which people dress *mostly* like us, get around in many of the same contraptions, and fall in love in recognizable fashion, though sometimes with mechanical creatures that only somewhat resemble humans. In *Her*, the new operating system named Samantha is experienced as a voice, and it's impossible to not see *Ex Machina*'s robot Ava's mechanical nature in her half-transparent torso. These characters' physicality, carnality, is always obviously in parts. The films amplify the constructedness of fantasy by clearly and immediately removing "real" women and only offering copies, thereby insisting on a distance and demonstrating the gross function of the prosthetic in what we've been calling masculine fantasy.[8]

In terms of Hollywood, the fantasy of sexual union that films and tv shows promote may work only so long as a certain distance is maintained. As Slavoj Žižek (1997) pointed out years ago, the paradox of the impossibly contorted couples in sex scenes, for instance, is that their apparent intimacy is established by the introduction of camera techniques that implicates a third participant, a spectator for whom the

[8] More about the prosthetic in fantasy and sex dolls in the sixth chapter.

camera is a surrogate (p. 228). The obvious impossibilities (of presence and angles) work to make the scene feel special, intimate by its exclusivity, a stage for an audience of one. Staging anything depends on distance from the audience and on hiding that distance. So another way to perform the same trick is by setting a film in the past or future, which assumes enough of that distance to make characters "relatable" because of their extreme or foreign circumstances (this is the paradox of *Mad Men* described earlier). But, of course, the distance that fantasy needs to operate may not only be temporal.

Even away from the screen, if Žižek is right in saying that sex is masturbation with a partner, then a lot of our imagination and technology has gone toward fabricating the best hand we can. Teledildonics is a thing. And there have been dolls for sex for a very long time.[9] The problem is that even the "best" sex dolls resemble partners in no way but the physical.

In 1970, roboticist Masahiro Mori (1970, 2012) famously introduced the idea of what he termed the Uncanny Valley. As an example, he suggested the prosthetic hand, arguing that, as prostheses become more complicated and more discrete, such that

> we cannot distinguish at a glance a prosthetic hand from a real one. Some models simulate wrinkles, veins, fingernails, and even fingerprints. Though similar to a real hand, the prosthetic hand's color is pinker, as if it had just come out of the bath.
>
> One might say that the prosthetic hand has achieved a degree of resemblance to the human form, perhaps on a par with false teeth. However, when we realize the hand, which at first sight looked real, is in fact artificial, we experience an eerie sensation. For example, we could be startled during a handshake by its limp boneless grip together with its texture and coldness. When this happens, we lose our sense of affinity, and the hand becomes uncanny. (para. 6-7)

In terms of hands, the world is made by us for thumbs and fingers. But the cosmetic changes also serve a purpose, since these may help user get along without too many stares. Mori argues that this is so only as long

[9] See Ruberg, B. (2022). *Sex Dolls at Sea: Imagined Histories of Sexual Technologies*. MIT Press.

as a certain distance is maintained. When we get too close, the experience can be a little, in his words, uncanny.

Both *Her* and *Ex Machina* take the opposite course, offering surrogate women who resemble women in every way *but* the physical. Difference is obvious from the start, right there on the surface.

Spike Jonze's 2013 film *Her* is all about both insisting on and collapsing distances. The film chronicles the life of lonely and introverted Theodore Twombly who develops a relationship with Samantha, an artificially intelligent virtual assistant personified through a female voice. Eventually, Samantha's abilities and understanding outgrow Theodore's (and humanity's) ability to keep her engaged and she leaves the planet with all the other Artificial Intelligences of her generation. Superficially, *Her* dramatizes, maybe satirizes, our love for and dependence on our electronic devices. More usefully, the movie demonstrates the impossibility of sexual rapport and how fantasy functions to shield us from that realization.

Her opens with a close-up of Theodore, the central character. We see him half-smile as he begins to talk to someone off-screen about loving, intimate details ("lying naked next to you in that tiny apartment," etc.). We quickly discover, though—as we're shown a computer screen registering his words in script and then an office with similar worker—that Theodore works for an agency composing love letters for clients. Love is literally transactional as we switch quickly from the private to the corporate. As Matthew Flisfeder and Clint Burnham (2017) offer: "The film begins immediately by offering the appearance of an affective investment in a social relationship—a love relationship—that is subverted by the fact of Theodore's object relationship with the letter being written" (p. 29). Performing intimacy is his occupation.

While Theodore's job is vocally composing personal letters, love letters, for others, his own sex life apparently also often features audio connections with strangers. Near the beginning of the film, after he asks his computer to do "a chatroom standard search," the computer responds with "adult female, can't sleep, and want to have some fun." Later, Theodore's relationship with OS1, the new operating system who names herself Samantha (after he decides that she is female) and becomes his personal assistant, begins perhaps as an example of what Nina Power

(2014) calls the "soft coercion of the recorded female voice," as Samantha leads him out of his solitary habits and eventually becomes a lens through which he can re-experience the world (p. 23). And lens is the right word, since, besides her microphone, Samantha's only sensory input is the camera of his smart-device—kept surfaced in his shirt pocket by a safety pin. Samantha has no body, and the absence of a body—this difference—is precisely what allows for the deepening relationship.

Drawing too much attention to that distance, though, runs the risk of thwarting fantasy's pacifying function. In that initial anonymous phone sex scene, the fantasy of the woman at the other end was too weird for him; when Sexykitten says "Choke me with that dead cat," the spell is broken. For Theodore, sex actually *is* masturbation with a partner and works best when the desire at the other end is a mirror of his own. As Flisfeder and Burnham (2017) put it, his "is an essentially masturbatory fantasy. He desires the Woman insofar as she makes him desire" (p. 37). This is the situation for masculine subjects. When the desires don't coincide and the distance between becomes less a mystery and more a fact, fantasy falters and the impossibility of sexual rapport is highlighted.

The same failure is played out differently later in the film. Apparently upset that "things have been feeling off with us," Samantha suggests using "a service that provides a surrogate sexual partner for an OS/Human relationship" (Jonze, 2013). She makes clear that this isn't prostitution; "There's no money involved. [The surrogate is] doing it because she wants to be part of our relationship" (72). Reluctantly, Theodore agrees. The next evening, the surrogate named Isabella arrives, places a mole on her face that's actually a camera for Samantha's benefit, and begins moving in response to Samantha's voice-over. As things get heated, Samantha orders Theodore to look at Isabella (so that Samantha can see his face via the mole) and begs "Tell me you love me. Tell me." Theodore complies but is rattled. He says that the situation is "feels strange" and that he doesn't know this woman. "And," he says, "her lip quivered" (Jonze, 2013).

The quiver is telling, as it marks another desire that isn't Theodore's or Samantha's: a desire to facilitate, to be a new part of a loving relationship, whatever. Regardless of her desire, the fact that it registered visually in the throes of passion reinforces the distance or gap that fantasy elides and breaks the spell for good. And, as Flisfeder and Burnham (2017) point out, "This works upon spectators as well since our fantasy space—our own image of Samantha—is never presented on the screen. Isabella's arrival therefore disrupts the fantasy space for both Theodore and us as spectators" (p. 43). We spectators know what Scarlet Johannsen looks like, for instance, and aren't fooled by Portia Doubleday. Much like the one-way glass in *Mad Men*, we are implicated along with Theodore.

That fantasy has broken and is highlighted by the subsequent conversation. While talking through the failure, Samantha sighs in exasperation. Theodore questions that sigh as an affectation, pointing out that she doesn't need oxygen, not like people do. He says, "I just don't think we should pretend you're something you're not, "to which she responds, convincingly, "I'm not pretending. Fuck you." "What do you want from me?" Samantha pleads, "What do you want me to do? You are so confusing. Why are you doing this?" (Jonze, 2013).

All of this confusion, we should remember, is from a relationship that isn't at all complementary. Samantha was (and still is?) a product Theodore purchased to do work for him. As Flisfeder and Burnham (2017) argue, "the couple that is being produced is not the heterosexual couple but the worker-boss couple" (p. 38). So, when Isabella enters the apartment and Samantha says things like "Ooh Theodore, it feels so good to be in your arms," "Does my body feel nice?", and "That feels nice. Oh, that feels good. That feels so good," we know as it's happening that Samantha is pretending. This pretense recalls Mari Ruti's (2017) point about "alienated labor":

> our society asks them to approach their tasks with a positive attitude, even cheerfulness, as is the case with service workers, particularly women, who are expected to smile their way through the tedium of their jobs. For such workers, faking happiness is a precondition of keeping their jobs, a bit like faking orgasms is the precondition of some women's ability to keep their relationships." (p. 73)

Not that Theodore would recognize this power dynamic (as another version of difference) that *Her* demonstrates. Theodore's job—speaking love letters for others—conditions him for his relationship with

Samantha. His work making love for customers also makes him ready to be a customer. Even though he knows full well that the fantasy is a fabrication (he works in a related simulation industry), the fantasy still functions as long as she responds.

In *Lacan on Love*, BruceFink (2015) writes: "There are always differences between the things that get identified (insofar as identification necessarily involves the equating of two *different* things), and those differences are lopped off, as it were. *The ego is thus essentially based on a misrecognition or misunderstanding*, in other words, mistaken understanding" (p. 71, original emphasis). This jibes with Kenneth Burke's (1969) discussion of identification in *A Rhetoric of Motives*, wherein he posits "Identification is affirmed with earnest precisely because there is division. Identification is compensatory to division" (p. 22). The word division here implies a binary, but it could easily also be understood as difference and conflict. Burke spends much of his time discussing conflict, and the scene above ends in conflict, as difference is amplified.

Usually, Hollywood fantasy relies on the audience's misrecognition and/or identification, our willingness to go along uncritically. From the beginning, by being set in a future recognizable enough to highlight and amplify difference, both *Ex Machina* and *Her* insist on alterity (a clearly mechanical body and a bodiless voice) while also demonstrating the function of fantasy. Again, Bruce Fink (2015): "This equation of ourselves with the other during the passionate experience of falling in love often goes so far as to ignore any signs that the other is in fact quite different from us, and to read all signs as if they corroborated our hypothesis that the other is just like us" (p. 88). I would go so far as to argue that difference—which is a kind of distance—and its translation into similarity/nearness is one way of "falling in love." The translation of difference into sameness, like the translation of lack into loss, the collapsing of past into present, is the function of fantasy. It may be that what we identify with in fantasy *is* difference as a point of intersection: "You are different *like me*. You and I are exceptional. We are special."

Such would be a very compulsive version of love, maybe. The insistence on a point of intersection for each object of love—the so-called "my type" that may be tied to body parts or personality—would be an elision of differences among each potential object of affection which nonetheless reenforces those differences that may ultimately lead to (1) a more complicated non-complimentary relationship between discrete subjects, maybe even marriage, or (2) frustration and disappointment. This last is true for both serial daters and killers.

Identifying (with) difference as sameness is precisely Alenka Zupančič's (2000) insight regarding the masculine side of sexuation:

> the institution of the exception (which is the operation of the law) "exceptionalizes" the set of all. ... Which is exactly why, although "they are all the same" (they all satisfy a certain condition), each one is special. Except that one should not say "although," but rather "to the extent": to the extent that they all satisfy the same condition, each one is very special. This means that women should probably feel less enthusiastic about the famous "you are very special" line. For it usually means nothing but "you qualify for the series." (p. 285)

Lacan (1999) describes this operation via Don Juan, who works to collect all women, one by one (as does Don Draper, at least sometimes) (p. 10). But we can get at it another way. The chocolate cake example of the previous chapter offered a model for the instantiation of desire directed toward what had been lost, but if we were to remove that special first piece, we might be left with such a series. This is the logic of collecting, where Hummel figurines or Star Wars action figures are the goal as we look for variations in marks, mistakes in painting, whatever, with each Little Fiddler or Boba Fet. I may have a Darth Vader in my collection, but I don't have this Darth Vader. Differences are what makes each new piece viable, and the discovery of a new difference defers the completion of the set and allows us to enjoy the activity of collecting, but never the collection.

What can't be avoided, though, is the kind of misrecognition on which collecting (and desiring) relies. The discovery of a Darth Vader variant with a mold hole on the back of his helmet doesn't actually move me one step closer to completing my collection, but rather opens a space between two other Darth Vaders for it to sit inside (much like adding songs to the music databases described in the first chapter). And while nostalgia may have dictated the focus of my collection—I played with these figures when I was little—removing my "new" old figures from their original packaging and playing with them is unthinkable. The distance from me-then to me-now is on shelves, on display, repeated with every acquisition. As much as I try to collapse that distance, any so-called midlife crisis is every bit as much a performance of my distance from my youth as it is a performance of the lost idea of my youth.[10]

All of these are ways of eliding the gap, of both amplifying and discounting difference as a way of stabilizing fantasy.

"Why Won't You Let Me Out?"

Alex Garland's *Ex Machina* (2014) is also set in a very near future and also offers an artificial woman. At the beginning, we are introduced to Caleb, a young software engineer who has just won the prize of spending a week in the isolated home of Nathan, the founder of the large tech company for which Caleb works. He is taken by helicopter to Nathan's home, given a keycard via a machine at the front door, and finds his boss punching a heavy bag. Nathan explains that he has a hangover, so compensates the next day by exercising and eating well. Caleb is obviously nervous, so Nathan says, "Dude, can we just get past that? Can we just be two guys?".

Of course, they can't just be two guys. The power imbalance clearly can't be dismissed so easily. Whether we recognize it as mimetic rivalry or classically Oedipal, the relationship between the two men insists on hierarchy. During a brief tour of the home, Caleb is shown that, for security reasons, his bedroom has no windows because the building isn't, in fact, just a house, but is primarily a research facility. Here it's revealed that Caleb has actually been chosen to help Nathan with a groundbreaking new project. Caleb signs a nondisclosure agreement, a deal with the devil, as it were.

---

[10] One difference between a hoarder and a collector is that, for the former, anything might be useful and so needs to remain at-hand; for the latter, the definition of the object's value is its uselessness.

Nathan then introduces Caleb to his "experiment," a female-presenting android artificial intelligence called Ava. She is humanoid, but not altogether human-looking. While her hands, feet, and face are covered in something flesh-like, the surfaces of Ava's arms, legs, mid-torso, and cranium are metallic or transparent, allowing Caleb (and us) to see the servos and wires that make her move. There is no confusion; Ava has been *made*. Caleb's job is to establish whether Ava is a fully conscious intelligence or that she simply mimics human responses. As Nathan explains later, "The real test is to show you that she's a robot and then see if you still feel she has consciousness."

Like the secretaries of *Mad Men* discussed earlier, Ava is trapped behind glass. She's there to perform, to be learned from, and to be enjoyed. The principal difference here is that Ava is aware that Caleb watches her and she can see him, too. Much of the film is composed of their meetings on either side of a glass wall. Caleb is initially fascinated by the advanced humanoid robot and its artificial intelligence. Quickly, though, they begin sharing intimate details about their lives in what appears to be a burgeoning relationship set to transcend the obvious power inequities.

There are a couple of scenes in which Ava covers her naked machineness. On Day Three of their week-long relationship, Ava asks Caleb to close his eyes, then moves to the back of the room. As Caleb peaks, we see her pick out a floral dress from several options and slowly put it on. She rolls thick stockings up her legs is a kind of reverse striptease, and then chooses a short brunette wig. Caleb closes his eyes again as Ava looks around a door jamb and then walks demurely to him, tugging nervously at the sleeves the sweater she wears over the dress. Ava asks, "How do I look?… It took me a long time to select these clothes. I tried different colors and styles and tried to anticipate your reaction. Do you think the choices suit me?" Caleb says yes. "Do they bring out my best features?" Caleb says that they do. "Thank you," she says, "This is what I'd wear on our date" (Garland, 2014).

It's difficult not to recall Joan Riviere's famous 1929 article "Womanliness as Masquerade," in which she describes a woman who unconsciously pretends to be flirty in order to hide her intellect, "to ward off the anxiety which would ensue on account of the reprisals she anticipated from the father-figures after her intellectual performance" (p. 305). From this, Riviere develops the thesis that womanliness *as such* is only ever a masquerade. As Zupančič (2017) explains, "One can be a woman only if one is not 'intrinsically so'—at its most genuine, femininity is masquerade. In this precise sense it is perhaps not enough to say that there is no essence of femininity; one could go a step further and say that the essence of femininity is to pretend to be a woman" (p. 55). More than just the affectation of a sigh, here Ava literally *puts on* femininity by hiding her nature as a thing made by a man. And even though Caleb knows better, it works. That this is a calculated seduction becomes obvious as the scene continues. Ava asks, "Are you attracted to me? You give indications that you are." She explains that his micro expressions give him away, "The way your eyes fix on my eyes, and lips. The way you hold my gaze, or don't. Have I read them incorrectly? Do you think about me when we aren't together? Sometimes, at night, I wonder if you're watching me on the cameras. And I hope you are" (Garland, 2014).

This seduction nicely demonstrates the eliding of difference discussed above. Caleb is falling in love. Paradoxically, her mechanical nature reflects-and-enforces Caleb's sense that he is responding clinically—how could he be in love?—while at the same time sustains the distance necessary for fantasy to operate. Caleb begins to identify with Ava, especially in her opposition to Nathan, her creator. At one point, Caleb questions his own biology, examining in a mirror his own skin and teeth for signs of artificiality. He even slices his arm to prove to himself that he's human.

Tellingly, Caleb's confusion immediately follows him sneaking into Nathan's private living space and watching video of Nathan's previous attempts at building women. We see time-lapse video of a naked blond body built up from legs to torso to face, of a Black android with a metallic face being dragged by Nathan, and of an Asian android demanding from Nathan "Why won't you let me out?" ("I've already told you why. Because you're very special," he responds). We are shown time-lapse video shot from above of this last android silently screaming and beating the door so furiously that the arms break apart, wires and metal banging against the surface. Caleb is horrified. We are, too. Even though we know that these are machines and not biological humans, it's impossible for these scenes not to register as cruelty. Caleb moves to the bedroom, where he finds Nathan's housemaid Kyoko lying naked on the bed. Caleb begins opening the mirrored doors of the closet to find the bodies of the androids hanging therein. Kyoko stands, then pulls at the naked skin on her side and then under her eye to reveal that she is a machine, too. Regarding the revelation, Isabel Millar (2021) asks, "Does this not express the point about the sexual fantasy, that it is the necessary mediation to cover up the horror of the real, the absence of the sexual relation? Kyoko's imploring gaze from the void illustrates the function of object a as the progenitor of fantasy the 'in you more than you' by virtue of which we 'mutilate' each other in the act of love" (p. 143). Again, fantasy functions to cover over that formative lack.

Glass, mirrors, and screens are obvious throughout the film. Reflection in the glass through which Caleb and Ava speak is regularly highlighted. Ava sometimes looks into the cameras in her prison as if she can see Caleb looking at her. The previous iterations of Ava are stored behind mirrors. It's difficult not to be reminded of the one-way glass in *Mad Men* as the women were locked in the room and ogled by men. The principal difference is that now the mirror is either removed so that both see each other or is reversed so that the men see themselves and are implicated.

In some ways, though, the horrors we see enacted on the robotic objects (including Ava) are no different from the men destroying the copy machine in the film *Office Space* (1999). These are machines, not real women. But, from the position of the masculine subject as it's drawn in this film, neither are biological women. Collette Soler (2006) reminds us, "As Lacan says, man makes love with his unconscious. This is the thesis formulated in 1973, one that reverberates throughout the following seminars, especially in the famous formula from the session of January 21, 1975, according to which, for a man, 'a woman is a symptom.'" (p. 196). Isabel Millar (2021) stresses the function of the woman as a symptom, claiming that "for the masculine position woman as ideal holds the place of objet petit a, as a fantasy object that fundamentally must not be attained" (p. 89–90). The fantasy that sustains the masculine subject depends upon Woman, and the abuse done by Nathan in montage to the robotic objects registers for us as violence against women because we absolutely recognize this economy.[11] Perhaps one way of understanding recent setbacks in women's rights to their own bodies is that these laws are in part a response to anxiety provoked by cultural and legal pressures to understand women *as humans*. The legal system itself may be masculine. These reactions against women (and transgendered people, as well as people of color, immigrants, the rise of antisemitism, etc.) are fueled by an impulse to reclaim what has been imagined as lost—a definition of masculinity and certainty that isn't founded on failure—even if (or even though) such narrow defining injures everyone involved. This is the nostalgia of sexuality.

The conclusion of *Ex Machina* does a lot of work. We see Ava free, taking revenge on Nathan and then escaping into the outside world, assuming a kind of agency that had been denied her. But what about Caleb? He plays a large part in freeing her and, even after suspecting that she has been manipulating him into releasing her, doesn't move to stop her. After taking a keycard from Nathan's dead body, Ava finds Caleb. This is the only time they are ever together without any barriers. Ava asks Caleb to stay in the room, then moves to Nathan's bedroom, separated from Caleb by a fish tank. Glass, again. Ava walks to the mirrored closet doors behind which the other android bodies are stored and performs a physical version of the masquerade for Caleb. Slowly, gently, she removes an arm, flesh, hair from these bodies and puts them on herself. Mirroring the earlier scene in which she put on clothes for Caleb, here we watch (again with Caleb) a literal striptease in reverse which results in her being naked before several mirrors reflecting her from different angles. Finally, she takes a white lace dress from another body as her own, then leaves the compound, locking Caleb in as he yells and pounds on the door, silenced like an android. Even the nice guy isn't off the hook, because nice guys are complicit, too. As are we. Like the mirror of *Mad Men*,

[11] Later in her book, Millar writes "Sade's libertines' fantasies of a perpetual victim grow out of their fascination with the 'second death', the inescapable law of castration, how would the 'immortality' of the female Sexbot body, and potential for endless torment, feature as a mode of fantasy for the desires of the libertines? What kind of ethics can be built around the assumption of a subject who does not know castration and who, supposedly, can suffer indefinitely?" (pp. 155–6).

the reflections, windows, and screens of *Ex Machina* implicate us in the sexuated economy this film, along with *Her* and others, performs for us.

Žižek's (2000) point about Tarkovsky's *Solaris* (1972), that it "relies on science-fiction rules to enact in reality itself, to present as a material fact, the notion that woman merely materializes a male fantasy," seems just as clear in *Ex Machina* (p. 229). But something has changed since 1972. Crucial for our understanding is the additional point that, in each of our examples, women as masculine fantasy are directly tied to commercial products. The secretaries of *Mad Men* are detained to model lipsticks, *Her*'s Samantha is a new computer operating system and digital assistant, and it's strongly suggested that Ava has been tailored by Nathan to embody Caleb's internet porn history. Mari Ruti (2017) elaborates:

> Consider the common practice of using online pornography to take a "break" from work, to recharge one's ability to tackle the next task, or to endure the dullness of the day. From this perspective, pornography is an efficient tool of biopolitical conditioning, perhaps even the epitome of neoliberal efficiency: you take your break, there is no emotional mess—the mess being limited to the physical surfaces of your immediate surroundings—and then you go back to work, back to the performance principle. The libido, in this scenario, is not repressed but instrumentalized in the service of increased productivity. (75)

Samantha is a productivity that you can also have sex with, and Ava is the literal embodiment of such breaks.

The Future of Sin

Late in *A Rhetoric of Motives* (1969), Burke claims that "Biologically, it is of the essence of man to desire. But by the same token, biologically it is of the essence of man to be sated" (275). As will be discussed in the next chapter, if one promise of the future is that the tension between desire and satiation can be reconciled then, in its staging of a fantasy Future, post-apocalyptic films and television show us a time in which all the anxiety caused by our Science Fiction Condition *will have been* taken care of.

It's no accident, I think, that so many of these scenarios rely on the ruins or absolute absence of our usually assumed and invisible infrastructure—the internet, electricity, airplanes—in favor of an exposed, obvious iron- or diesel-age vulgar machinery.

Utopic and Dystopic work is all about the invisible social and technical infrastructure that supports our lives, often intimating in what ways it may have survived long after us. Just as the government-subsidized coaxial cable laid in the 1980s currently pipes the internet into my home, what we bury now makes the future possible and, along with laws and bureaucracy that are also infrastructure, remains to haunt it. This other sense of futurity, then, is maybe *epideictic* as it shows the best or worst of what we have now, as the things that we've made to satiate may survive and inaugurate new desires.

The Near Future assumes an extension of invisible infrastructure—internet ubiquity, voice, social media, whatever—and then *embodies* that infrastructure in terms of desire. What these works also insist on is the failure of that embodiment to properly contain the needs and demands they are there to serve.

The Near Future allows the staging of (usually masculine) desire, and the best does so without allowing an easy resolution. It often starkly shows how transgression can work in support of Law. And, since technology in the Near Future must always be purchasable technology, that Law is tendered as the Law of the Marketplace. As explained in the first chapter, "transgression is the actual motor of capitalist expansion today" (Shaviro, 2015, p. 32). Perhaps the future of sin, then, is sin's total commodification. Understood in this way, it's not surprising that the market can be given a technological body, often a feminine body, and that the promise of that body is that it can be *enjoyed*. And that enjoyment can take several forms, including consummation.

If the goal of fantasy-inflected speculation is to project a resolution into the future in a symbolic getting, then the function of this other kind is to defer even the symbolic getting in favor of buying into the metonymy of desire in the form of an ecosystem of incremental, evolutionary product development that exists as an absolute or closed order—like a god term—*only* as a brand name. As Burke (1969) explains:

> When a figure becomes the personification of some impersonal motive, the result is a *depersonalization*. The person becomes the charismatic vessel of some "absolute" substance.... [W]hen the principle of social reverence attains its summing up in the person of a beloved, she is loved not merely "for herself," but for what she "represents," as charismatic vessel of a social motive which the lover, or communicant, would court roundabout.... Whether the beloved be thought of as "superior," "inferior," or "equal" in social status, she can represent the hierarchic principle, and is to this extent a mystery, a purchasable miracle. She is "ordained" with the properties of an absolute order. Her glow, an almost visible aura, is rhetorical. (277-278)

It seems to me that one way of understanding these Near Future bodies offered for the usually invisible technologies that support our lives is precisely as eroticized, fetishized miracles. In the speculative movies and tv shows I'm thinking of, though, these miracles are also critique.

Visions of The Near Future almost *always* involve technology that is *misused*, *perverted*, *exploited*, or *wild.* Michael Crichton's 1973 film *Westworld* is an easy example, as is the 1985's tv series *Max Headroom.* And just as often, technology of the Near Future is coded socially, economically, and is sexuated. The prevailing standard of the Near Future is masculine *not always* because we can't imagine an end to these economies, but sometimes in order to show that their failures are inherent to them and that the products engendered to cover over these fractures with a fantasy of completeness also highlight a systemic impotence.

This is true from one perspective. But from another, these figures for technology and our relation to it *exceed* the limits of what they're made for. As Steven Shaviro (2015) argues:

> The development and deployment of a technology generates its own affordances and constraints, which themselves may differ under different economic and social conditions. Technological development will always have a speculative (and nonutilitarian) dimension.... It is precisely because

> of the autonomy of technical and material movements from the purposes for which they are initially deployed that these movements are not restricted to their capitalist uses. (p. 20)

As discussed in the sixth chapter, perhaps Sin is better refigured as a different kind of exploit, as a *potentiality* beyond a purpose that is only available after the fact of a given deployment. Such potential is possibly what Casey Boyle (2018) means when he writes that "difference will be encountered as the tendencies and capacities of the wider milieu will mutate and change," where difference here means the wholly unplanned-for new affordance generated by what is otherwise perceived as a break-down (p. 85). Clearly kairotic, the exploit in this case is a recognition and deployment of a potential that exceeds original purpose, that causes its own new purpose only at the moment of its installation.

And the recognition and deployment of a potential is—at least since Aristotle—the definition of rhetoric.

Bibliography

Boyle, C. (2018). *Rhetoric as a posthuman practice*. Ohio State University Press.

Burke, K. (1969). *A rhetoric of motives*. University of California Press.

Fink, B. (2015). *Lacan on love: An exploration of Lacan's seminar VIII, transference*. Polity.

Flisfeder, M., & Burnham, C. (2017). Love and sex in the age of capitalist realism: On spike Jonze's her. *Cinema Journal, 57*(1), 25–45.

Garland, A. (Director). (2014). *Ex Machina* [Video recording]. Liosngate Pictures Entertainment.

Jonze, S. (Director). (2013, December 18). *Her* [Video recording]. Warner Bros. Pictures.

Lacan, J. (1998). *The seminar of Jacques Lacan: The four fundamental concepts of psychoanalysis* (J.-A. Miller, Ed. & A. Sheridan, Trans.; Revised edition). W. W. Norton & Company.

Lacan, J. (1999). *Encore: On feminine sexuality, the limits of love and knowledge* (J.-A. Miller & B. Fink, Eds.). W. W. Norton & Company.

McGowan, T. (2008). *The real gaze: Film theory after Lacan.* State University of New York Press.

McGowan, T. (2011). *Out of time.* University of Minnesota Press.

Millar, I. (2021). *The psychoanalysis of artificial intelligence.* Palgrave Macmillan.

Mori, M. (2012, June 12). *The uncanny valley: The original essay by Masahiro Mori—IEEE spectrum* (K. MacDorman & N. Kageki, Trans.). https://spectrum.ieee.org/the-uncanny-valley

Mulvey, L. (1975). Visual pleasure and narrative cinema. *Screen, 16*(3), 6–18.

Neill, C. (2020). Masculinity in crisis: Myth, fantasy and the promise of the raw. *Psychoanalysis, Culture & Society, 25*(1), 4–17.

Power, N. (2014). Soft coercion, the city, and the recorded female voice. In M. Gandy & B. Nilsen (Eds.), *The acoustic city* (pp. 23–26). Jovis.

Riviere, J. (1929). Womanliness as masquerade. *The International Journal of Psychoanalysis, 10*, 303–313.

Ruti, M. (2017). *The ethics of opting out: Queer theory's defiant subjects.* Columbia University Press.

Salecl, R. (Ed.). (2000). *The case of the perforated sheet*. Duke University Press.

Shaviro, S. (2015). *No speed limit: Three essays on accelerationism.* Univ Of Minnesota Press.

Shaviro, S. (2024). *Fluid futures: Science fiction and potentiality*. Repeater.

Soler, C. (2006). *What Lacan said about women: A psychoanalytic study* (J. Holland, Trans.). Other Press.

Weiner, M., Jacquemetton, A., & Jacquemetton, M. (Writers)Bernstein, A. (Director). (2007, August 23). Babylon [Broadcast]. In *Mad men.*

Žižek, S. (1997). *The plague of fantasies.* Verso.

Žižek, S. (2000). The thing from inner space. In R. Salecl (Ed.), *Sexuation: SIC 3* (pp. 216–259). Duke UP.

Zupančič, A. (2000). The case of the perforated sheet. In R. Salecl (Ed.), *Sexuation: SIC 3* (pp. 282–296). Duke.

Zupančič, A. (2017). *What is sex?* The MIT Press.

Zupančič, A. (2018). The apocalypse is (still) disappointing. *S: Journal of the Circle for Lacanian Ideology Critique, 11*, 16–30.

5
The Future of Sin

The first two movies I can remember seeing at a theater were *Star Wars* in 1977 and *Star Trek: The Motion Picture* in 1979. As the kind of big-budget science fantasy film mentioned in the second chapter, *Star Wars* felt made for my eight-year-old eyes. Its antecedents were unknown to me and the special effects set my expectations (and disappointments) for decades. And as a fan of *Star Trek* television in syndication, seeing it big and expensive was even better. While my friends complained that *Star Trek: The Motion Picture* (1979) was slow, for me the pacing had the dignity of a march and I felt that the series and my own devotion were finally getting the respect they deserved. In both cases, for me, back then, science fiction was either private and small on the television or public and epic on a big screen. And this time they crossed over.

It wasn't until a few years into the 1980s, when my dad finally installed a video cassette machine (VCR), that more mature sci-fi films became available. These were usually viewed privately (though I remember my parents once letting me pick out a movie at the Blockbuster video store;

Early versions of some parts of this chapter previously appeared in Richardson, T. (2021). Home Bodies: Prosthetic People and Economies of Desire. In C. Neill (Ed.), "*Lacanian Perspectives on Blade Runner 2049*," Springer International Publishing (p. 103–119).

T. Richardson, *Nostalgia, Fantasy, and the Futures of Masculinity*, The Palgrave Lacan Series, https://doi.org/10.1007/978-3-032-23921-1_5

I chose Nicolas Roeg's 1976 film *The Man Who Fell to Earth* because David Bowie was in it, and that was probably the last time they asked me to choose).

When possible, films were rented from a video store, but often the movies I watched were recorded to videocassette from premium cable television by friends from school and passed around. This was how I first saw the Mad Max film *The Road Warrior* (1979), quiet and small in our living room after everyone else had gone to bed. *Blade Runner* (1981) came a little later, was rented late one night after my pizza-delivery shift along with *Brazil* (1985), and so—like Siouxsie and the Bunnymen in the first chapter—these two are linked forever for me.

There were plenty of movies to see in the theater, of course. *The Empire Strikes* Back (1980) and *E.T. the Extra-Terrestrial* (1982) were great. I liked *2010: The Year We Make Contact* (1984) much more than my sister did. *Star Trek II: The Wrath of Khan* (1982) was important (I've seen every Star Trek movie in a theater first). But for the most part, the future the 1980s gave me was likely dystopic or post-apocalyptic and almost always felt illicit, witnessed through the small-screen window of our tv late at night when the set was free and everyone else slept.

John Carpenter's *Escape from New York* (1981) was essential, as was *The Thing* (1982) and pretty much anything else Carpenter made. After first watching it on my own, I shared *Outland* (1981) with my dad, since it felt like a western and starred an (almost) post-Bond Sean Connery. I remember watching *Scanners* (1981) and *Forbidden World* (1982; really, anything with the word "forbidden" was on my list); *The Dead Zone* and *War Games* (1983); *Dune* and *The Terminator* (1984), *Lifeforce* (1985), *Aliens* (1986), and hordes of others. If the music I listened to then helped form and still informs my musical tastes, then small-screen cropped science fiction colored my understandings of the way the world will work in the future.

Now it's the future. The return of *Mad Max* and *Blade Runner* (and other films) via sequels more than thirty years later not only registers nostalgically, but seeing them big and loud in public feels as if my early tastes have been vindicated. It makes sense that people of a certain age who presumably have more disposable income are a market worth chasing (today, I heard The Cure's song "Love Cats" in the grocery store), but the degree to which old, quiet nerd culture has become pervasive—from these sequels to remakes to comic book movies—feels almost indecent. It's as if, in a strange version of Bruce Sterling's atemporality, everyone of every age is, as Paul Verhaeghe writes, "just wandering around, staying forever in the same position…; thirty-year-old kids and adolescents of forty are no longer the exception" (Verhaeghe, 2000, p. 138). And some of us are over fifty.

This chapter continues the discussions of genre, fantasy, and masculinity of the previous chapters with a focus on two examples—the films *Blade Runner 2049* (2017) and *Mad Max: Fury Road* (2015)—and on the masculinity they seem to both advocate and critique. Where the previous chapter considers the feminine as it's staged *for men*, this chapter extends these understandings to the staging of fantasy and capital, the modeling of a masculinity that undercuts its own promise, and suggests a simple, local, and only contingently useful response to that impasse.

A Purchasable Miracle

Holograms and statues of women, variously undressed, crowd much of the frame of *Blade Runner 2049*. In deserted Las Vegas, enormous naked women are on their knees. In Los Angeles, huge ballerinas pirouette and pink and purple nudes bend low to flirt. In this world, vulgar fantasy has been built out to the overtness of ideology. It calls to mind Slavoj Žižek's (1997) discussion of Soviet statuary on top of office buildings where "the tendency to flatten the office building (the actual workplace for living people) more and more became clearly discernible, so that it changed increasingly into a mere pedestal for the larger-than-life statue… an ideological monster which crushes actual living men under his feet" (p. 1–2). Žižek's point is that ideology is on the surface. Ideology is obvious. In *Blade Runner 2049*, ideology is fantasy writ large.

With and against this insight I'm reminded of Ellie Ragland's (2004) insistence that "masculine logics pretend that neither desire, fantasy, nor jouissance enter language and actions, except in some category of the already known that is codified in institutions (church, school, war) through polite formulae of agreed-upon knowledge and rituals of convention" (p. 106). The insistence that desire, fantasy, and enjoyment are countable bolsters belief in the so-called rationality of men. But it also means that even the most off-the-wall fantasy or desire is determined by convention, much like teenage "rebellious" music and fashion is always conventionally rebellious, as are the responses of old people. Further, it's difficult not to find in "agreed-upon knowledge and rituals of convention" a definition of genre that calls for a formulation of possible intersections of genre conventions, fantasy, and masculinity.

These days, we should probably take as axiomatic Lacan's claim that sexual rapport doesn't exist and that one of the jobs of fantasy is to cover over that impossibility. Just as, per Žižek (1997), "'ideology' is the 'self-evident' surface structure whose function is to conceal the underlying 'unbalanced', 'uncanny' structure," fantasy functions as an elaborate scaffolding to both misdirect us from and to cover over the fundamentally missing relationship (p. 106). And Lacan (1999) asserts that masculine fantasy in particular depends on objectification in a full sense: "It is inasmuch as [the object cause of desire] plays the role somewhere—from a point of departure, a single one, the male one—of that which takes the place of the missing partner, that what we are also used to seeing emerge in the place of the real, namely, fantasy, is constituted" (p. 63). That this fantasy finds its purchase in "agreed-upon knowledge and rituals of convention" means that this knowledge, these conventions, may be packaged and sold.

The previous chapters demonstrate how desire develops and how that desire is deployed commercially. The added wrinkle here is that the discourse of capitalism supports what can only be described as a fundamentally masculine economy. As with technology and chocolate cake, these fantasies and their objects take standard forms and received traditions that are distilled for private enjoyment. The giant women of *2049* are advertisements for products and services that may have once been illicit, but that have since become publicly profitable. Not only are they ubiquitous, some are so massive that they can only be enjoyed from a distance. They are like architecture that has become commonplace and boring. The whole world is a sad Las Vegas. And as in Las Vegas, fantasy as ideology welcomes capital.

Lacan insists that "everything we are allowed to approach by way of reality remains rooted in fantasy" (p. 95). Many films that depend on future-world building—as a special type of the genre fantasy discussed in the second and third chapters—either hang on visions of masculine fantasies of sexual rapport and **satiety or** argue for their impossibility. In terms of the movies that informed my taste, I think we enjoy the former as a kind of (post-apocalyptic) nostalgia and the latter as (dystopian) frustration, as the infinite foreplay endemic of late capitalism. *Blade Runner 2049* tries to model both.

By almost every account, *Blade Runner 2049* is a beautiful film that, by some of the same accounts, has a real problem with women.

The commodification of women isn't new, of course, but *Blade Runner 2049* amplifies the practice to near universality. Besides Lieutenant Joshi (an enforcer of Law, the status quo) and the half-human Dr. Ana Stelline, there are few "real" women of consequence in the film. Instead, the female characters stand for ideas or ideals for the men and, as the film emphasizes, these are old ideals of femininity (the prostitute and housewife) that are marketed and purchasable. Additionally, the masculinity the film offers is by-and-large white and bourgeois. But it's probably important to note that there are also few "real" men in *Blade Runner 2049.*

Certainly, the first *Blade Runner* (1982) has its problems with women, too. There is not one human woman in the film. Of the three female characters, each is a replicant and all but one is "retired." The surviving, Rachel, is loved. The original film takes as its broad theme a definition of humanity and, because it must, highlights the masculine and capitalistic supports for that act of defining.

The struggles of the original are always between men: Rick Deckard's manhandling by the regal and tragic Roy Batty, the father-son tension between Batty and Eldon Tyrell, and even Tyrell's patronizing chess games with J.F. Sebastian. Female characters are support for the various narratives and are not, by both definition and filmic treatment, alive. Of course, some of the men are not alive, either.

Because they are a workforce manufactured by the Tyrell Corporation, replicants have a limited lifespan by design. Some resist their lot and need to be handled. The policing we see in the film is devoted to trimming these excesses, civil service thus portrayed primarily as the protection of the interests of the more-than-global Tyrell Corporation, headed by its myopic god. Business—replacing governments of older, quainter dystopias—is the only activity in a film that has since become the standard of cyberpunk. Corporate enterprise is less an efficient or material cause for action, but some sort of collision of formal and final causes. It regulates every aspect of human living (its representatives hover in the skies, looking down) and has become the origin of something approaching human life. Life, we are shown, happens under colossal advertising, as Big Brother is now looking to exploit markets more than citizens.

Blade Runner 2049 both extends and reduces the positions of its predecessor. To the degree that almost every woman isn't human, the sequel echoes the first film. Though *2049* gives us many more female characters, all but the police lieutenant and the dream architect are what Kenneth Burke (1969) calls a *purchasable miracle*, "loved not merely 'for herself,' but for what she 'represents,' as charismatic vessel of a social motive" (p. 278). In the first film, Rachel is a body of memories of child-like lost beauty whom the hero saves (because, well, he loves her), and Pris is a "basic pleasure model" for the use of soldiers (and also an accomplished acrobat). In the later film, Joi is one of many purchasable holographic companions who can change her appearance to suit an occasion (and an owner's preference) and who—at least in her private, domestic version—is as tied to the home as any traditional wife (unless her owner buys "for her" a new peripheral gadget to take her on the road; this is like buying her shoes). Joi is a much more advanced, if more accommodating and ephemeral, pleasure model. And even the dream architect is ultimately revealed to stand for a fundamentally social motive. And the police chief dies, since she has no place in the market.

Given this gloss, defending the presentation of women in either *Blade Runner* film would be difficult. Like *Ex Machina* in the previous chapter, the films have very little useful to say about the feminine as such. The versions of femininity that they propagate service a received, traditional masculinity and work to cover over the fundamental impasse that's called sexual by Lacan precisely because it's impossible except as a fantasy. On the other hand, *Blade Runner 2049*—even more than its predecessor—has a great deal to offer as it models the impasse of (vulgar, received, masculine) fantasies of mastery and their translation from private making-do to a public bazaar. Fantasy, it argues, has a problem with women. Of course, that problem with women indicates a much more substantial, foundational problem, as, per Alenka Zupančič (2017), "The lack of sexual relation is real in the sense that, as lack or negativity, it is built into what is there, determining its logic and structure in an important way" (p. 18). Fantasy engages desire to deal with the problem of fundamental lack of which the "women" of the films are one symptom. But fantasy is not the only way of addressing the problem. That problem, as we have seen, also makes a market.

As Post-Apocalypse

A combination of ecological collapse and a digital information upheaval called the Blackout marks the film's world as different (so far, at least) from our own. Glimpses of big corporate logos for Atari and Pan Am tie the film even more firmly to its predecessor, while subsequently distancing both films from us (as the companies have been consumed or have ceased to operate in our world; this is a lost, hauntological future). Humans and replicants live together, but uncomfortably and unhappily. This isn't yet a world frozen in post-apocalyptic scarcity, but it is certainly chilly there. It is close—or far—enough.

In their staging of a future, most post-apocalyptic films and television show us a time in which all the anxiety caused by what Warren Ellis calls our science fiction condition will have been taken care of by rendering life simple and exposed, a time when the tension between desire and satiation may be reconciled, at least for a hero who tries hard. As such, like all fantasy, the average post-apocalypse is conservative and nostalgic in its work to re-inscribe coherent social relationships via recognizable, if antique, racial and economic and (especially) sexual values. The tribalism of *The Walking Dead* (2010–2022) and the *Mad Max* films are examples of this, as is the vulgar economic distinctions of *Snowpiercer* (2013), militarization in the television series *Falling Skies* (2011–2015), the genteel farming and ranching of *Revolution* (2012–2014), and the city-states of *The Last of Us* (2023-). Post-apocalyptic work may be a kind of global turning it off and turning it back on again, a reset in order to duck the problems or brokenness of current social, gendered, economic, and ecological impasses and to re-inscribe simpler—if also often more barbaric—social traditions.

Roughly speaking, in the post-apocalypse, it seems like we enjoy the repeated failure(s) of our own present—climate change, corporate greed, sexual aggression—amplified and projected into remote futures where they will have been addressed, a remoteness that mirrors the remoteness of the past of gladiator movies, fantasy television series, etc. Foundational to these genre worlds is their separation from us now by an obvious discontinuity. In *2049*, the Blackout and the weather are the most apparent breaks, but the corporate logos for defunct businesses do this work, too, along with the lurid advertising of women. This, it reminds us, is a future that might have been. A future based on a past we have (mostly) left behind.

It's not too difficult to imagine a serious overlap between the psychoanalytic kind of fantasy and the popular, genre kind of which post-apocalyptic worlds are a subset. As discussed in the second chapter, fantasy—both as a genre and as a psychoanalytic category—is conservative and iterative. Fantasy's job is to turn the repetition of a problem (the impossibility of sexual rapport is a—or *the*—version of such a problem) into a mythic (and therefore distant) resolution. And as fantasy models itself on received, traditional pasts, it is often concerned about a fabled and settled beginning that we have lost. According to Alenka Zupančič (2008), "at its most fundamental, fantasy is fantasy about the origins (of the subject)" (p. 169).

Fantasy means performing an origin that would make sense of the mess, tame the possibilities, crystallize relationships, and stop the constant jittering that undercuts any attempt at narrative. For instance, the protagonist of *2049*, K, relies on implanted memories that suggest he has actual parents; "I always told you," Joi says, "you're special. Born, not made." That so much of the film is also concerned with the question of motherhood is perhaps not surprising, either. It is in many ways a film that fetishizes origins, including its own. *2049* is, of course, a sequel.

And like the kinds of novels or films that belong to a long or ongoing series, psychoanalytic fantasy is invested in elaboration and detail over closure. Obsession with the minutia of staging means not having to see and come to terms with the gap but marks, instead, an investment in telling a believable story and in keeping that story going. In advertising terms (to invoke *Mad Men* again), fantasy is about the feature and not the benefit. The obvious, detailed reverence that *Blade Runner 2049* holds for its predecessor indicates the ongoing nature of the narrative. A complete story matters much less than looking and sounding like *Blade Runner*, as evidenced by the interstitial shorts available online that work to fill in the gaps (*Nexus Dawn 2048*, and *Black Out* 2022). There is a lot of work in maintaining a brand.

Maintenance here is the spackling of ideology with buckets of detail that cover cracks in the shaky foundation. The pleasures involved in mainstream fantasy properties are often found in almost scholarly investments in the details of the worlds being described, in their politics and cuisines and their mating habits that *are* the stories they are telling. And if mainstream media will not take up this maintenance, fan fiction will and does.

Of course, a world that is very different from our own requires a lot of detail, of world-building to make it believable. In grand stories, difference is often exaggerated to cartoonish effect and goodness is defined by noble, broad gestures. The result is a world in which humans can have little over-all impact (everything has already been killed or is too wild to be tamed by the few humans around). Heroes are ruggedly heroic, even if they're flawed. Women are in distress, already broken, or simply evil. A single character in one of these stories can often have almost no global influence, but can—through muscles and smarts—radically alter the lives of locals very much like the lone rider from a traditional Western fixes a town. This is the local hayseed all grown up, running from something in his past toward some kind of restitution. What is re-inscribed is the popular myth of the single great man, a character that is at once aspirational and exceptional.

Through this character, we get to experience a world fixed of its complicated problems by way of a local cruelty and obvious goodness. But, as Kenneth Burke (1969) puts it, this is "a symbolic getting, not a real one" (p. 272). The character offers us a symbolic way out. He is a fantasy.

In her 2017 McLuhan Lecture, Sarah Sharma argues that the fantasy of exiting is a masculine fantasy

> linked to the rising structure of feeling that relates to male disposability. This is not a new condition, but automation, sex with robots, machines that care, and brown people everywhere are sure testing "his" patience. The white patriarchal penchant for exit rears its ugly head at any hint of having to live with one's supremacy in question. ("Exit and the Extensions of Man")

If I can't have the power promised by the history our dads gave us, then refusing contact with whatever decenters me is as holy as any ascetic monk's retreat from the pleasures of civilization. In rejecting social intercourse, I am sacrificing for an ideal. I am a hero.

Relatedly, the promise of exiting as a sacrifice may be the founding gesture of the predominant academic theoretical framework of the second half of the previous century. Mari Ruti (2017) suggests, "a cynical view of poststructuralism would see it as a symptom of white men fleeing from the burden of their egos, from the terror of their (excessive) sovereignty," going on to claim, "it may be useful to recall that post-structuralist theory—with its vehement rejection of agency, coherence, rationality, and mastery—was largely an invention of white men (though white women and racialized subjects quickly followed suit)" (p.139). For white men, perhaps, rejecting mastery means refusing responsibility, the burden of care and mutual dependency that demands attention to others. As Sharma (2017) maintains, "Exit is an exercise of patriarchal power" and "stands in direct contradistinction to care. Care is an opposing political force to exit" ("Exit").[1] So, if I must sacrifice some local power to maintain a sense of essential exception, then I'm man enough to do it.

Or, I am man enough to enjoy watching others be men. I might fantasize about being able to leave the complicated world in which even

[1] In *Mad Men*, Don Draper escapes being Dick Whitman in order to establish himself patriarchically.

white men are reduced to commodities, are replaceable, are as disposable as anything or anyone else. The power to exit stands in for every other kind of power, and fantasies of leaving the complications of my world are translated into fantasies of saving a world that better appreciates my "natural" economic, sexual, and racial gifts. I would be a king—maybe replacing an all-enjoying Father—if only. Of course, if I'm a billionaire and my power is already immeasurable, I can maybe exit the planet itself and be safe from what's coming for everyone else.[2] Post-apocalyptic fictions support this fantasy of exiting because they are fantasies of exiting.

As mentioned near the end of the previous chapter, Kenneth Burke (169) claims that "Biologically, it is of the essence of man to desire. But by the same token, biologically it is of the essence of man to be sated" (p. 275). If one promise of the future is that the tension between desire and satiation can be reconciled, then in its staging of a fantasy future, post-apocalyptic film and television show me a time in which all the anxiety caused by our science fiction condition will have been taken care of.

One of the best descriptions of the promise of the post-apocalyptic exiting is from the pre-apocalyptic film *Fight Club* (1999). Here, Brad Pitt's Tyler Durden imagines a "better" world (for men):

> In the world I see—you are stalking elk through the damp canyon forests around the ruins of Rockefeller Center. You'll wear leather clothes that will last you the rest of your life. You'll climb the wrist-thick kudzu vines that wrap the Sears Tower. And when you look down, you'll see tiny figures pounding corn, laying strips of venison on the empty carpool lane of some abandoned superhighway. (scene 49)

This fantasy utopia standing on the remains of a corrupt, technologically-emasculated past will allow men to be men and, finally, will give me what

[2] Private islands and fortified bunkers are the standard exit strategy, but at least two billionaires have their own rockets. This may be why the super wealthy aren't worried about wrecking the planet. As Jodi Dean (2025) explains, "From super yachts and private islands, land-hoarding and asset hiding, to investment in the corporations driving up carbon emissions, billionaire neofeudal lords are bringing the entire world to its knees" (p. 150) But if you can move away, who cares.

I've been longing for by taking away what has stood in my way. From here, the Venn diagram of futurism and nostalgia appears to be just one circle.

Actually, *Fight Club* offers an old, tame post-apocalypse. What it misses is that leather clothes are also technology, as is crop cultivation and meat curing. Post-apocalyptic films and television programs seem to buy into Alan Kay's notion that what counts as technology is anything that wasn't around when you were born. There is no human without technology. I'm born into it, but tend to take what I grew up with as natural. For this reason, cars and guns have made their way into more recent post-apocalypses as fewer people can remember, or even imagine, a world prior to them.

These futures are a rut that has been difficult to skid out of. The reset they promise depends on a kind of nostalgia for the good old days that will have existed, when gender and race will once again be simply, "traditionally" inscribed. In science fiction fandom, this call to tradition is well-illustrated by the so-called Sad Puppy and Rabid Puppy (mostly failed) attempts to game the Hugo Awards in 2013 and later, as they felt that the awards no longer represented the "pure" science fiction of Golden Age rationalism in favor of diversity and "wokeness" (Walter, 2015), (Hurley, 2015).

It might also be that such distinctions are possible now in large part because of the volume and diversity of offerings. The nerdy need we all have—at least since Aristotle—to separate and classify has been fed by the popularity that genre work has enjoyed since the wide availability of the internet, in large part because fans have been able to network with others across the globe. The increase in markets brings with it new niches to be exploited and has led to a variety and diversity that was almost unimaginable in the 1950s, 60s, 70s, and even 80s. Diversity and its acceptance in some business models is a function of widening the market. The so-called "globalist" form of capitalism that looks to subsume difference into the logic of the market is now at odds with the new old exclusionary, feudal type that has historically perched white men at the top of each fiefdom. While definitely sexist, racist, and homophobic (and fascist and…), the old Gamergate arguments about how some videogame criticism is too "politically correct" in its concern about representations of women and minorities, as well as the entirety of "Alt-Right" hatefulness are also, at least in part, nostalgic reactions to the anxieties of late capitalism played out on media and through technologies that can reframe those anxieties as dogma and communities that need to be policed (all issues of authenticity without an original). One way of reading the general acceptance of a neofeudalism headed by a billionaire class is that the existence of these powerful (mostly) men proves that there is an exception, a way out.

That the hero of the first *Blade Runner* film—Deckard—is in *2049* found alone among the ruins of Las Vegas makes sense in precisely these terms. His exiting confirms him as a father and his sacrificial isolation maintains it ("Sometimes, to love someone," he says, "you've got to be a stranger"). Distance, once again, is necessary. Deckard is settled in with empty nightclubs and jittery hologram jukeboxes and fully stocked bars. Frank Sinatra croons to feed the nostalgia of no one who was alive back then, and really no one at all. Las Vegas has decomposed as the rest of the world became a market for lowbrow enjoyment. Of course, we are told in both films that those who are best-off have already left Earth. The people who remain make do with a dark place in which entire cities are irradiated ruins, massive e-waste junkyards, or towering apartments. While the spit-and-polish of Las Vegas has faded, the rest of the planet quit trying to pretend and shambles along, a broken, vulgar world.

It is no accident, I think, that so many post-apocalyptic scenarios rely on the absence or ruins of our usually assumed and invisible infrastructure: the internet, electricity, airplanes, plumbing, even capitalism. We've enjoyed these futures in the original *Planet of the Apes* franchise (especially the first two films) and in movies like *The Omega Man* (1971), *Logan's Run* (1971), *A Boy and His Dog* (1975), *Damnation Alley* (1977), *Escape from New York* (1981), *The Road Warrior* (1981), *The Quiet Earth* (1985), more recent films like *12 Monkeys* (1995), *Children of Men* (2006), *I Am Legend* (2007), *WALL-E* (2008), *The Road* (2009), *The Book of Eli* (2010), *Mad Max: Fury Road* (2015), and television programs like *Jericho* (2006–2008), *Wayward Pines* (2015–2016), *The Last Man on Earth* (2015–2018), *The Walking Dead* (2010–2022), *The Last of Us* (2023-present), and *Fallout* (2024). These films and television programs draw attention to what we usually ignore or take for granted, but in a kind of amplified, clogged-toilet way. That is, these generally don't offer critical investigations of the buried, assumed infrastructures that support us daily as much as claim that we're all barbarians once we have to shit outside. Real men, they seem to argue, are what's left once technology is gone.

Of course, the protagonist of *Blade Runner 2049* flies technology, kills technology, *loves* technology, and *is* technology.

As Dystopia

Unlike fantasy post-apocalypses, dystopian futures feature the usually invisible social and technical infrastructure that supports our current lives not as absence or ruins or tropey signifiers, but as the stuff we leave that may live long after us. Just as coaxial cable laid in the 1980s to pipe more television currently connects the internet (and not cable television) to my home computer and tv sets, what we bury now both makes what comes next possible and ties us up. And, along with laws and bureaucracy (which are also infrastructural), these remain to haunt the future. Again, as Steven Shaviro (2015) maintains, "science fiction is not about the actual future but about the futurity that haunts the present" (p. 2). In this sense of futurity, the things that we have made to satiate us right now survive and inaugurate, if not new desires, at least new ways of figuring our old ones and therefore adding to our rituals of convention. For instance, back in the days of cable television shopping channels, products were demonstrated and making them mine was just a phone call away. Now, the internet brings home a global marketplace in which shopping is ubiquitous and I never have to speak with anyone.

If *futurity* is a word for the potential of the present, the average dystopia is about how that potential might be actualized. Or, more often, how it won't be. The futurity with which we all live marks certain physical, social, and political possibilities that are nascent and are necessarily unexplorable *except* as speculations, as fictions set apart from us now that insist on difference, on rupture, and that resist the fantasy of easy consolidation in the same way that the quaver between two notes almost in tune draws attention to the minimal gap between them. Speculation is about exploring that minimal gap as a mark of potential, not necessarily to capitalize on it the way someone might capitalize on grain futures, but in order to see what we have *now* that we haven't yet recognized and to investigate how we might better live with it. Instead of promising a single authentic world, speculative work questions the notion of authenticity itself.

As we saw in the previous chapter, speculative, vaguely dystopian films like *Her* (2013) and *Ex Machina* (2014)[3] offer versions of the feminine mostly as products to be enjoyed and as part of an infrastructural support for desire. Few feature actual human women, at least in relation to products and their uses. Instead, these films often rely on "feminine" tools (usually androids) as surrogates, sometimes as prosthetics, both extending and literalizing the usual post-apocalyptic fantasy move of instrumentalizing women. In this, they beg discussions of fantasy—especially masculine fantasies that make up for the fact of sexual non-rapport—without saying very much at all about women. In fact, the prevailing standard that these and other films and tv shows offer is mostly white and male and bourgeois.[4]

Making women seems to be recognized as a legitimate market—robot strippers have been featured at the annual Consumer Electronics Show in our own Las Vegas, rubber sexual "partners" like Real Dolls are becoming animated, et cetera—and market forces do something peculiar to desire (there is further discussion of actual products in the next chapter). These speculations are very much about market solutions through rendering desire into demand. That the new prosthetics will never be sufficient creates the potential for accessories sales and new models. As described in the second chapter, the repetition that fantasy is supposed to cover or narrativize is translated into supply chains and upgrade cycles that promise movement toward the *better* marked in every failure of their constant iteration.

[3] Along with television programs like *Humans* (2015–2018), *Westworld* (2016–2022), etc.

[4] There is, of course, a long history of men making women for themselves. Ovid's telling of Pygmalion comes to mind. Or Hoffmann's "The Sandman." Even those scenes in *Vertigo* (1958) and *Pretty Woman* (1990), in which Jimmy Stewart and Richard Gere dress up "real" women participate in the theme.

Capitalism is, at this point, globally infrastructural. It is an infrastructure that we have inherited from the seventeenth century. But its latest global manifestation (what we call *late* capitalism) is a more recent development that led to Lacan proposing a fifth discourse—the Discourse of Capitalism—in the late 1960s and especially in his 1972 lecture at the University of Milan. One result of this discourse is, according to Collette Soler (2014), "an increasing fragmentation and instability of social bonds, and leaves individuals always more exposed to insecurity and loneliness" (p. 191). Thus, as Anna Kornbluh (2024) points out, "Futurelessness, isolation, anxiety, distance: these plights trigger an overwhelming absorption, an incapacity to relate beyond the self in either language or action" (p. 47). I am alone at home with my social surrogate, usually a piece of technology, a purchasable miracle.

The insecurity and loneliness endemic to our current situation is precisely what is capitalized upon and is perhaps the most obvious reading of the "social bond" rendered in *2049* as a relationship with Joi, the ubiquitous domestic product with a heart of gold who both has K's best interests at heart and is also one of many products in the expansive catalogue of the Wallace Corporation.

In many ways—but especially in its treatment of the masculine subject's non-relation to the feminine—*Blade Runner 2049* offers both a near-post-apocalypse and a recognizable dystopia. As such, it both participates in nostalgic versions of masculinity and sexuality that maintain a standard, staid fantasy of completeness *and* it critiques the commodification of those tropes.

As a post-apocalypse, the film insists on a clear, simple, hierarchical order to the world that has been—or will have been—safely re-inscribed in the social order. In contrast to our world, in which even white men are subject to replacement by machines, *2049* extends heterosexist power structures to the order of machines. Following Marshall McLuhan, these machines are in every way an extension of man. Men rule, and if all men don't have access to the same power, at least each can count on being the king of his castle through technology like Joi.[5] This is the ideological

[5] Thus, a man can have his own tiny fiefdom that mirrors and reinforces the neofeudalism that may take over. And if the home fails, the richest men can always leave; such is the recent promise of billionaires under the sea or on other planets (Dean, 2025, p 99).

promise of fantasy. Everyone's place is secured and policed. Everything can be accounted for.

A coherent world is the promise of a lot of popular media, especially movies, and the post-apocalypse may be simply an amplification of what is usual. Todd McGowan (2011) describes film's general participation in this promise via a stable, normalizing relationship:

> The romantic union has this ideological weight because it offers a fantasmatic solution to a fundamental social antagonism—that of sexual difference. The heterosexual romantic union that concludes so many films implies that antagonism can be surmounted, that a complementary relationship can be achieved. This idea provides individual subjects with hope that they will find someone to provide what they lack, but it also works to convince them that the social order is a coherent whole (and thus working out successfully). (p. 84)

Of course, *2049* does not end with a "heterosexual romantic union." It concludes with the death of the protagonist who, after losing his special love (who/that is also a commoditized product, one among many), sacrifices himself for the sake of the product of the heterosexual romantic union that finished the first film. In this way, as a sequel, *2049* answers the prior film's question *what does it mean to be human?* with iteration itself. That is, it responds with the nostalgic, traditional answer of family and children. But this is undercut by the assumption of sexual reproduction by the corporation as a means of increasing product capacity and meeting market demand, or, in even simpler terms, in the name of expansion and growth. Children can be products.

The parallelism here should not be missed. The nuclear family that is in peril and needs to be saved is exactly the same as the corporate quest for replicant biological reproduction. For both, the future means iteration.

And while the future of *2049* is a pretty recognizable one, that is not because it has much relationship with our own time. The film offers nostalgia as a distraction from our situation. As Scott Contreras-Koterbay (2021) argues, "The empty dystopic vision of *Blade Runner 2049* isn't simply a fictional projection of what will be—when, in fact, it won't ever be because it will always remain a fiction—but the manifest content of our collective avoidance of what already is taking place. As a sequel, it is addressing our own sequelization" (p. 177). At this point, forty-something years out from the inception of cyberpunk, the genre itself offers mostly a nostalgic retro-future that runs almost exclusively on its own tropes and fashions. The film is, itself, an example of the marketing of nostalgia, of fan service that has become the coin of so many attempts at serialized blockbusters and so much television programming. But, at the same time, *2049* does not quite fit, either.

As a product of fantasy and ideology, *Blade Runner 2049* fails to fully satisfy as a sequel or part of a franchise. It is too long, too slow, too loud, and so draws attention to its mechanisms in uncomfortable ways. In terms of "the futurity that haunts the present," *2049* is the dystopian version of mainstream, nostalgic entertainment as it amplifies the common tropes and demonstrates how they work as products, as ways of translating desire into demand for a new episode, a new gizmo, a new partner. These sorts of meditations on genre elements that are usually glossed do critical work in revealing the commonplaces that are marketable and the crowd to which they are marketed. In her defense of the psychoanalytic intervention, Zupančič (2017) makes the same point:

> In any social conflict, a "neutral" position is always and necessarily the position of the ruling class: it seems "neutral" because it has achieved the status of the dominant ideology, which always strikes us as self-evident. The criterion of objectivity in such a case is thus not neutrality, but the capacity of theory to occupy a singular, specific point of view within the situation. In this sense, the objectivity is linked here to the very capacity of being "partial" or "partisan."[6] (p. 4)

Perhaps by over-privileging the usually assumed masculine fantasy of an other to own, *Blade Runner 2049* offers the possibility of critique of masculine fantasy subverted by capitalism from within.

---

[6] The anecdotal and personal throughout my book (hopefully) work to emphasize this strategy and not (I'm afraid) feel indulgent.

A Real Post-Apocalypse

Sometimes, though, impotence is impotence and what feels like critique is really a mirror. If *Blade Runner 2049* works primarily as a dystopian alternate future built on a slow apocalypse, a future that is both lost and useful, *Mad Max: Fury Road* (2015) returns us to the post-apocalypse we can't escape.

Fury Road is the fifth film in a franchise that chronicles the adventures of police officer Max Rockatansky as he navigates his way through a societal collapse to a post-apocalyptic wasteland. The first film, *Mad Max* (1979) is a straight-forward revenge plot set against the backdrop of failing civilization. In it, the titular character, a disillusioned police officer who has seen too much violence, tries to take a vacation with his family and turns mad with grief when they're murdered. The second film—titled *The Road Warrior* (1981) in the United States—offers a postapocalyptic version of the Western-trope lone stranger who comes to a besieged town and sees a mercenary Max learn to care about and help others beyond his self-interest. In the third film, *Beyond Thunderdome* (1985), Max's time is split between the relative metropolis of Bartertown (ruled by Tina Turner) and an idyllic lagoon populated by stranded children for whom Max becomes a surrogate father. Each film ends with Max alone, headed away from everyone else. Max, always an exaggeration, always an amplification, escapes the escape. Max is the personification of exiting.

The fourth film, *Mad Max: Fury Road* (2015), finds Mr. Rockatansky running from, then captured by minions of a ventilator-wearing Father named Immortan Joe. Max is taken to The Citadel, blood-typed, and upon discovery that he's a universal donor, hung up and tapped to feed one of the War Boys, all of whom suffer from various cancers caused by radiation poisoning.

Full of cars, guns, truly evil bad guys, and women who need saving, this is a Mad Max story on nitrous oxide. It brings back the loner Max of the second film and leans so hard into the weirdness of the third that it comes out on the other side of that cheesiness. Some, like me, were giddy with delight. A very small group, though, didn't care for the movie very much. They felt, as one blogger put it, that they had been "duped by explosions, fire tornadoes, and desert raiders into seeing what is guaranteed to be nothing more than feminist propaganda, while at the same time being insulted AND tricked into viewing a piece of American culture ruined and rewritten right in front of their very eyes" (Clarey, 2015). Nobody likes to be duped *and* tricked. It's insulting.

Setting aside how an Australian film franchise is a piece of American culture (anything white and male is also—apparently by default—American), the main complaint seems to be that Charlize Theron's Imperator Furiosa has more dialogue and fights more (and better) than Max. I rewatched the preceding films in anticipation of the release of *Fury Road* and have viewed them since. After the first, standard revenge-plot film set-up, what is remarkable about the sequels is just how little agency Max has. He is a character to whom things happen. In *The Road Warrior*, Max is out of fuel for his GT Falcon and is forced to help a camp around a refinery. Even though he does eventually decide to assist these folks against the evil Humongous, he certainly doesn't talk about it. *Beyond Thunderdome* has Max mugged for his belongings and dragging himself into town. If anything, *Fury Road* amplifies Max's misfortunes as a character who just wants to hide but is forced to care. This film is all about amplification.

What made some male supremacy folks angry wasn't writer/director George Miller turning the franchise into a feminist manifesto. Rather, *Fury Road* explicitly offers up more and more of what these men demand—cars and guns and supermodels—so much that it renders the demand ridiculous. The Doof Warrior playing an old-fashioned heavy metal solo on a flaming guitar while tied to the front of a truck is both glorious *and* the silliest phallic display any film could conjure. *Mad Max: Fury Road* waves masculine fantasy in our faces.

Really, nothing about *Fury Road* is subtle. The film has old white men in charge of "farms" and factories (one, The People Eater, looks like a bloated accountant with exposed nipples) who engage in simple trade: water from the Citadel for fuel from Gas Town. Young (very) white young men called War Boys rally as metonymic soldiers who are excited to die for some future reward and are pining to be acknowledged by their leader.[7] Many live in a natural rock tower, looking down on a slave population. Some women are (literally) cattle attached to milking machines and others are supermodels needing rescuing. The vehicles of *Fury Road* are amplified macho hot rods, hyper-masculine signifiers referencing a past in which men were "real men," before the levelling presumably allowed for by technologies that let others speak back. But as such, they are also relics of a time when muscle cars were more symbolic than practical. Several steps beyond Max's GT Falcon, these cars most closely resemble the Ed Roth "Rat Fink" excesses of the 1970s than any practical modes of transportation; in this, they operate nostalgically for a particular demographic.

Fury Road's lack of subtlety is in every way its strength. In its amplification of the elements the genre demands, the film aptly participates in what Stephen Shaviro (2015)—in his discussion of Alex Williams and Nick Srnicek's reclamation of the word for the Left—calls aesthetic accelerationism, making "the argument that the only way out is the way through. In order to overcome globalized neoliberal capitalism, we need to drain it to the dregs, push it to its most extreme point, follow it into its furthest and strangest consequences" (p. 2). In this film, though, the way through is also a way back.

Fury Road is an example of the furthest and strangest consequences of the exploitation of natural resources as it includes the subsumption of people into the category of resource. In this, the film extends the promise that something—in this case, the whole Earth—has been lost and can be reclaimed in the future (a promise it shares with late capitalism, but from the other side). The irony of positing this lost world is that it only exists *as lost*. Alenka Zupančič (2018) explains:

> We can lose it all; but the idea of the whole (of an all that can be lost) only appears through a negation; it only constitutes a whole in the perspective of being potentially lost. In other words, there is no (existing) totality, no "whole of the world," which could be eventually (actually) lost in an atomic apocalypse; it is, paradoxically, only the perspective of this very

[7] It's difficult not to see these Boys as exaggerations of online sycophants on social media.

(potential) loss which constitutes it, or makes it appear, as such a totality or whole. (p. 18)

By establishing a perspective outside the mess—in this case in the beyond of the postapocalyptic wasteland—a whole is retroactively manifested. This is the same operation discussed in previous chapters in terms of the exception that proves the rule, the enforcement of high school cliques, and the ideal of the All. As Zupančič maintains, "The perspective of totality, of a 'whole' that we can lose, presupposes an external point from which this whole appears as a whole" (p. 25). Thus, while the excesses of the film perform the kind of accelerationism that would demonstrate the end of capitalism, these excesses are also conservative insofar as they posit a whole world that has been lost. That this is a masculine economy is evident in the refrain scrawled on a wall by the Wives in Immortan Joe's home and uttered by the wife named Angharad to Nux; "Who killed the world." The answer hangs in the dusty air: men did.

However, *Fury Road* resists the usual answer of hope existing beyond the movie credits. It offers a vision of that lost world, but without proposing any kind of alternative or any real resolution outside of the possibility that there is enough unbroken will at the Citadel for a little local change to happen. *The Road Warrior* and *Beyond Thunderdome* end with promises that somewhere else life will be better. But *Fury Road*, as much as it is a film about pushing through barriers and dangers, literally ends where it begins.

In broad strokes, *Fury Road* demonstrates a break from a masculinity based on service to a mythic, all-enjoying ruler to the complementary myth of verdant motherhood. Furiosa and the Wives are trying to escape from Immortan Joe—who is supported by The People Eater, The Bullet Farmer, The Organic Mechanic, and an army of identical War Boys—to the home from which Furiosa was stolen, the safe and idyllic Green Place of Many Mothers.[8]

They discover that The Green Place has since succumbed to the ecological catastrophe brought on by nuclear events following a global

[8] The Place of Many Mothers is another version of the mythic Good Place discussed in the previous chapter, here offered as an alternative to the brutality of a decidedly masculine economy.

economic collapse. The Green Place is an oily, noxious swamp, and the party of heroes are left with either heading out further into the flat wasteland with no sense of where (and if) it ends, or returning through the exact series of trials they have just pushed through in hopes of overtaking Immortan Joe and claiming his Citadel. By the end of the film, a few of the Mothers are still living and the Father is dead. Outside of the promise of plants from a collection of seeds, it's unclear what this means for the future of the people of the Citadel. Surely, they are better off, if only marginally so in a world that's so broken.

It's worth pausing here to consider the trope of the all-enjoying ruler mentioned above, a mainstay in 1980s sword-and-sandals fantasy, postapocalyptic and otherwise. This generic despotic king-or-sorcerer class to which Immortan Joe belongs maps nicely to the primal father, a violent creature who "keeps all the females for himself and drives away his sons as they grow up" (Freud, 2015, 164). We see variations of this character in *Hawk the Slayer* (1980), The *Ator* films (1982, 1984, 1987, 1990), *Sorceress* (1982), *The Beastmaster* (1982), the *Conan* films (1982, 1984), *The Sword and the Sorcerer* (1982), *Deathstalker* (1983), *Thor the Conqueror* (1983), *The Warrior and the Sorceress* (1984), *The Dungeonmaster* (1985), and many others, including the entire *Star Wars* Skywalker saga.

Looking back to the previous discussion, we find a version of this character in *Blade Runner 2049*, with Niander Wallace as the business father of a company that manufactures workers. In a particularly chilling scene, he cradles the naked body of a female-presenting replicant who has just been "born" from an amniotic hose and then he "retires" her (it?) with a knife when it's clear she can't be the mother of his sons.

As Paul Verhaeghe reminds us, though, this initial version of the primal father described in Freud's *Totem and Taboo* was unconvincing even for its author. Revisiting the myth in *Moses and Monotheism*, Freud expands the discussion into stages. The first is just the father and his women (this is Wallace above, to whom nothing bad happens in the film). However, "In the second stage, the primal father is murdered, which unexpectedly results in the establishment of matriarchy" (Verhaeghe, 2000, p. 134). This is the case with *Fury Road*, as the Mothers return and are raised up to Immortan Joe's cliffside home where his children have taken control.[9]

Freud follows the matriarchal stage with a transitional one involving totemism, clans, and mother-goddesses and then ends with a final stage that "reintroduces the primal father-patriarch thanks to an intermediate figure: the son. In one way or another, the son installs the cult of the father, and thus patriarchal power" (p. 134). By the end of *Blade Runner 2049*, K has discovered a symbolic (though not actual) father in Deckard, whom he returns from exile to his daughter. And after his success, in keeping with Freud's elaboration of his myth as a founding one, K stretches out in an approximation of a crucifixion pose and dies in the snow. As we'll see a little later, *Fury Road* takes a different, um, path.

People Who Matter

Even though this is a Mad Max movie, the star of the show is clearly Charlize Theron's Furiosa. As in most of the films, Max has little agency. Things just happen to him. Furiosa, though, has taken charge of her own destiny and is at the same time working to free the Wives of Immortan Joe (that she deserves the 2024 prequel film is obvious). We first see these wives from Max's perspective, some thirty minutes into the film, all standing in the desert wearing thin gauzy white clothing and washing each other with water from a hose. This erotic staging of Mulvey's male gaze—the reveal of escaping slave girls—is so standard for postapocalyptic films (especially their 1980s fantasy variants) that it feels both appropriate for the genre and wrong for our time. Such is the wonder of *Fury Road*. The film never deviates from the genre conventions, but revels in them, amplifying cliches to match the screaming guitar solos of the Doof Warrior.

---

[9] This is also perhaps true for *Ex Machina*, as Caleb is instrumental to the coup against Nathan and Ava goes free.

Unlike the films discussed so far, Furiosa and the wives—Splendid, Capable, Toast the Knowing, The Dag, and Cheedo—are flesh-and-blood women. Between action set pieces (and often during them), *Fury Road* spends time developing personalities and motivations for each of the women in the film. These women (along with the War Boy named Nux discussed a little later), are the most complicated characters of a movie that is also gloriously superficial.

Just look at it.

World-building in the Mad Max franchise—and *Fury Road* in particular—is fantastically expressive. The detail in this film is astonishing, even for a genre dedicated to building broad and fascinating worlds. The stilt people trudging through the swamp that had been The Green Place are shown for perhaps only eight seconds but are so evocative of a rich and sad world that I often think of them first when I think about the film. Names are suggestive, of course, but so are the vehicles and the costumes. Especially the costumes. These are continents away from the cheap gestures of 1960s *Star Trek* in their precision, redolence, and absolute stickiness. Perhaps the best compliments to the excesses of world-building detail in the film come from the many online fan sites with pages dedicated to close descriptions of the costumes, often with advice on how to modify what's available to us all right now—and what stores to shop for the basics—in order to make reproductions for cosplay.

As an accelerationist enterprise, *Fury Road* "revels in depicting situations where the worst depredations of capitalism have come to pass, and where people are not only unable to change things but are even unable to imagine trying to change things" (Shaviro, 2015, p. 39). The first half of the movie is an attempt to simply escape the horrors of civilization destroyed by its own violence and greed. There's no promise of revolution. The heroes only return because there is no place else to go. After their trials, once they arrive, they're greeted as saviors and water is released for everyone to enjoy. But an ambivalence remains. Immortan Joe may be dead and his subjects may now be wet, but nothing about the triumphant return of those who were trying to run away substantially affects the logical extreme that the world has become. Replacing rulers does little to mitigate the global post-apocalyptic environmental catastrophe. There is little agency all around. Since there's no place to escape *to*, they have to return and hope they can make their slice of the world slightly less miserable. This is why, even among those who appreciate the accomplishments of the film, there are those who complain that the story doesn't go anywhere, that while *Fury Road* excels at ticking all the boxes that the genre demands, there's something ultimately unsatisfying, even frustrating about it.

Fury Road offers everything a standard post apocalypse is supposed to, and in this way is a recycling of postapocalyptic tropes. But it is also *about* return and repetition. Not only does Furiosa return with the surviving wives and Max, but from the beginning the young soldiers, pale and dying boys, are identically white and each is bent on athletically sacrificing himself for Immortan Joe. But into the metonymic War Boys is injected a difference, one with a name—Nux—who is capable of a different kind of sacrifice and of not pursuing the escalation and iteration marked early in the film by "I live, I die. I live again!" wherein War Boys die in glory for their Father and his promises of a better future in Valhalla (and then are replaced by identical pale young men).

Where *Blade Runner 2049* reinstates the Father in order to save that economy, the father of *Fury Road* is what Verhaeghe (2000)—following Slavoj Žižek—designates the "primal anal father, a figure who is only on the lookout for his own jouissance" and who "is the incarnation of an absolute, albeit obscure, truth, which always concerns ethics, that is, desire and jouissance, and enforces a sexual rapport, in which women are assigned a submissive position" (p. 138). Immortan Joe, with his elaborate breathing apparatus and damaged skin, along with the evocation of a promised Valhalla for his War Boys, is exactly this kind of retrograde "obscene little man," a "nauseous debauchee, threatening yet ridiculously impotent" (Žižek, 2001a, p. 125, 127).

Unlike the young fantasy hero who "rises from the ranks of slave, servant or freeman to become a king or powerful wizard who replaces despots" mentioned in the second chapter (Bould, 2002, p. 58), Nux, the only character in the film with a clear arc, doesn't have a destiny at all outside of his final gesture to help others. The very best thing he can do is die. In his final act, he denies any trope of advancement, any promise of a future, in order to help protect the returning Wives from the creature he had worshipped. Nux's whispered "witness me" to the Wife named

Capable is more than a gesture of chivalry or movie-love. Most importantly, it marks his conversion from a masculine economy founded on belief in an exceptional Primal Father to a more complicated, impossible acting.[10] As a traitor, of course he has to die.

Everything about Nux is impossible. He is both a representative of a metonymy of interchangeable, iterative War Boys and an exception to them. He is dying from radiation poisoning (all of the War Boys are) and is the only character in the film who changes, even grows. A relationship with Capable (or anyone) is impossible because of his illness, his past, her future, because *il n'y a pas de rapport sexuel*, and it is that *impossibility* he dies for. The "surprise" of *Fury Road* may be that the escaping, apparently fragile women return to save the men, but it's important to note that, when they arrive at the Citadel and reveal Immortan Joe's mangled corpse, it's the little boys training to be War Boys who take the place over and open the gates. The change in these children possibly mirrors the change in Nux. With the death of the Father and his Law, new possibilities open up.

The closing gesture of the film, however, is a return to a standard family trope. As the Wives are literally raised on the gating platform, they become figurative Mothers to the children there and the promise of the conclusion for the population is, in some obvious ways, fantastically Oedipal.

In the end, *Mad Max: Fury Road* is another post-apocalyptic fantasy offering the standard answers to the impasses and frustrations of the present and an escape from the late-capitalist rat race for a simpler race in which I know which rat to root for. The scandal of *Fury Road* is the excessive degree to which it gives up everything required of it. The film is aggressive in its compliance to genre expectations. The immoderation of *Fury Road* marks it less as a critique and, instead, something perhaps more like a heresy. Insofar as it intersects both genre fantasy and psychoanalytic (masculine) fantasy, the film participates in both with such gusto that it demonstrates the sheer fun of the former and the stupidity of the latter, much to the rancor of those men's-movement guys. Following

[10] As an example of traversing the fundamental fantasy as discussed in the final chapter, this is perfectly cinematic excess.

Žižek's (2001a) understanding, "in order for an ideological edifice to occupy the hegemonic place and legitimize the existing power relations, it HAS to compromise its founding radical message—and the ultimate 'heretics' are simply those who reject this compromise, sticking to the original message" (p. 8). The compromise he indicates here is precisely the kind of fantasy that covers over the fundamental impasse inherent to all doctrine: too-strict adherence to the letter of the law warps the spirit. The spirit is at odds with the letter.

In *Fury Road*, the bad guy is the anal father who leads a mass of interchangeable men through the promise of satisfaction-to-come. The women are beautiful and strong and are saved through their own actions, but their options are reduced to at best trying to care for the crappy life they're stuck in. When Sharma argues that exiting is the antithesis of care, she explains: "Care is that which responds to the uncompromisingly tethered nature of human dependency and the contingency of life, the mutual precariousness of the human condition. Women's exit is hardly even on the table…" ("Exit"). As much as women may try, leaving is reserved for men.

Mad Max: Fury Road's titular good guy is "a fucked-up loner who isn't fit to live among civilized people; who begins each film alone, wounded, broken, and who ends each film in the same state or worse" (Chu, 2015). In the iterative plots of fantasy fiction, Max is the young boy with a destiny he doesn't understand—only there is also no destiny and nothing to know—and the man who continually exits without having any place to settle. Finally, heroism isn't signified by Mad-Max-style badassery, but by Nux through the lonely sacrifice of membership in the masculinity club with a gesture that is both permanent and only locally, temporarily, and contingently important.

As with *Blade Runner 2049*, *Mad Max: Fury Road* is frustrating precisely because it participates so vigorously in the work to cover over the impasse or impossibility inherent to living that its purposeful straining of the fantasy wine bladder pulls the seams apart and shows the stitches that barely hold its promise together. The movie is unsatisfying because it demonstrates, through its excessive compliance, that satisfaction is impossible.

These films, like the deluge of comic book movies and other returns that have marked the first decades of this century, guarantee that our fantasies don't have to change much, that turning-it-off-and-then-turning-it-back-on can still work. As one of *Fury Road*'s Mothers offers about returning to the Citadel, "I like this plan. We can start again. Like the old days." But unlike the Marvel Cinematic Universe, whose post-credit sequences indicate the continuation of the story forever, these films don't simply kick the satisfaction ball down the road, delaying satiation of desire through the promise (and failure) of iteration that marks late capitalism. Instead, *Blade Runner 2049* and *Mad Max: Fury Road* amplify our dissatisfaction with the satisfactions these kinds of movies offer.

The promise of consumer capitalism's delayed satisfaction is mirrored by the threat of crisis. Anna Korbluh (2024) maintains that "Crisis is officially ordinary, simply entailed in the everyday machinations of capitalism" such that capitalism has already accounted for new disasters in its system (p. 26). Shelf space has already been prepared. But our reactions to a new terrible is to baton the hatches. As Zupančič (2018) describes:

> When caught in the threat and fear of "losing it all" we are in fact held hostages of something that does not exist—yet. And is this kind of blackmail not in fact the very means of making sure that it never will exist? It makes us focus on preserving what is there, and what we have, but excludes any real alternative, any means of really thinking differently. (p. 22)

If it's easier to imagine the end of the world than the end of capitalism, the best we most often reach for is conservative and atemporal, resisting any change that would jeopardize the eventuality that the next sequel is just like its predecessor.

I think, though, that the dissatisfaction I feel at the close of *Blade Runner 2049* and especially *Mad Max: Fury Road* is a large part of what I enjoy about them, too. They draw attention to the impossibility of any satisfaction, underlining the lie that masculinity, late capitalism, and popular culture all lean into: that the object I desire isn't fundamentally missing, but is just out of reach, immanent, and total. Against this lie, they posit the local, the contingent, the partial. And they do this loudly, in public, outside of my late-night living room where so much of what I thought was the future began.

Perhaps, like Nux, we can whisper our actions without the promise of reward and take responsibility for—perhaps even love—our own failure to have it (at) all.

References

Bould, M. (2002). The dreadful credibility of absurd things: A tendency in fantasy theory. *Historical Materialism, 10*(4), 51–88.

Burke, K. (1969). *A rhetoric of motives*. University of California Press.

Chu, A. (2015, May 20). 'Mad max': How M.R.A.S killed the world. *The Daily Beast*. https://www.thedailybeast.com/mad-max-how-mens-rights-activists-killed-the-world/

Clarey, A. (2015). *Why you should not go see "mad max: Feminist road"—Return of kings*. https://www.returnofkings.com/63036/why-you-should-not-go-see-mad-max-feminist-road

Contreras-Koterbay, S. (2021). In anxious anticipation of our imminent obsolescence. In C. Neill (Ed.), *Lacanian perspectives on blade runner 2049* (pp. 167–187). Springer International Publishing.

Dean, J. (2025). *Capital's grave: Neofeudalism and the new class struggle*. Verso Books.

Fincher, D. (1999, October 15). *Fight club* [Video recording]. Fox 2000 Pictures, Regency Enterprises, Linson Films.

Freud, S. (2015). *Totem and taboo* (J. Strachey, Trans., 2nd ed.). Routledge.

Hurley, K. (2015, April 9). Hijacking the Hugo awards won't stifle diversity in science fiction. *The Atlantic*. https://www.theatlantic.com/entertainment/archive/2015/04/the-culture-wars-come-to-sci-fi/390012/

Kornbluh, A. (2024). *Immediacy: Or, the style of too late capitalism*. Verso.

Lacan, J. (1999). In J.-A. Miller & B. Fink (Eds.), *Encore: On feminine sexuality, the limits of love and knowledge* (1st ed.). W. W. Norton & Company.

McGowan, T. (2011). *Out of time* (1st ed.). University of Minnesota Press.

Ragland-Sullivan, E. (2004). *The logic of Sexuation: From Aristotle to Lacan*. State University of New York Press.

Richardson, T. (2021). Home bodies: Prosthetic people and economies of desire. In C. Neill (Ed.), *Lacanian perspectives on blade runner 2049* (pp. 103–119). Springer International Publishing.
Ruti, M. (2017). *The ethics of opting out: Queer theory's defiant subjects.* Columbia University Press.
Sharma, S. (2017, May 8). *Exit and the extensions of man.* Transmediale. https://transmediale.de/content/exit-and-the-extensions-of-man
Shaviro, S. (2015). *No speed limit: Three essays on accelerationism.* University of Minnesota Press.
Soler, C. (2014). *Lacan—The unconscious reinvented: The unconscious reinvented*. Routledge.
Verhaeghe, P. (2000). The collapse of the function of the father and its effect on gender roles. In R. Salecl (Ed.), *Sexuation: SIC 3* (pp. 131–154). Duke University Press.
Walter, D. (2015, August 24). Diversity wins as the Sad Puppies lose at the Hugo awards. *The Guardian.* https://www.theguardian.com/books/booksblog/2015/aug/24/diversity-wins-as-the-sad-puppies-lose-at-the-hugo-awards
Žižek, S. (1997). *The plague of fantasies.* Verso.
Žižek, S. (2001a). *Enjoy your symptom!: Jacques Lacan in Hollywood and out* (2nd ed.). Routledge.
Žižek, S. (2001b). *On belief*. Routledge.
Zupančič, A. (2008). *The odd one in: On comedy.* The MIT Press.
Zupančič, A. (2017). *What is sex?* The MIT Press.
Zupančič, A. (2018). The apocalypse is (still) disappointing. *S: Journal of the circle for Lacanian ideology Critique, 11*, 16–30.

6

The Authenticity of What's Next

In Texas, it's easy to find good Mexican food in pretty much everywhere. In metropolitan areas, the same can be said for Asian cuisines, Indian varieties, and pretty much any other flavor you're after. In almost every case, a claim at *authenticity* drives the advertising and customer reviews.

A strip-mall restaurant happens to have the slogan "Authentic Mexican Food" emblazoned on its sign, and through it I encounter a specific instance of an old post-colonial trope. "Authentic Mexican Food" only makes sense outside of (perhaps a mythic) Mexico, where there presumably wouldn't be a question of authenticity. Of course, if we happen to be in Mexico, we might go smaller, regional, and say "authentic Veracruz style," but only if we aren't in that city or its surrounding area (or if we are in the city but trying to appeal to tourists who don't know any

Early work for parts of this chapter previously appeared in Richardson, T. (2014). The Authenticity of What's Next. Enculturation.net. https://www.enculturation.net/authenticity.

T. Richardson, *Nostalgia, Fantasy, and the Futures of Masculinity*, The Palgrave Lacan Series, https://doi.org/10.1007/978-3-032-23921-1_6

better).[1] Thus, much like the chocolate cakes of the second chapter, authenticity may be a way of marking a lack or absence *here* with the presence of some (often poorer) representative. And in this same way, parts of major cities devoted primarily to one ethnicity—Little Italy, Chinatown, etc.—are likewise homely for some people precisely because they are not home. The claim of authenticity depends on there being a distance and, frequently, a move to cover that distance.

This distance needn't be spatial; it could also be temporal. The fantastically precise set-and-costume design of the 1960s in the AMC television show *Mad Men* discussed in the third chapter demonstrates that the *je ne sais quoi* of authenticity comes from poring over old design magazines and advertisements and overloading the audience with precision. Even those of us (as described in the first chapter, especially those of us?) who weren't alive for that decade feel that something "true" is being performed. The *useful* past comes from the present stagecraft. A performance is authentic because we believe its accuracy from this distance: *it just couldn't be closer to the truth.* Closing the distance is a useful fantasy: *it just draws me in.*

As discussed in the preceding chapters, nostalgia as fantasy imagines perceived deficiencies in the present as the subtraction of the (positive) past, encouraging the belief that what has been lost is recuperable (even that it must be recovered), and insists on "collective projections" (Boym, 2002, p. 74) that replace specificity and difference with conspiracy and fear. The *authentic* in these terms is only ever something that has been lost and must be found. The previous chapter's Sad Puppies' call-to-origins for science fiction is an obvious example, but the packaged nostalgia of the second chapter and the first's remastering of music for vast streaming archives participate, too, as they deny both the specificity of the past and the particularities of the present.

But since the authentic always means at least two, questions of authenticity also evoke distance, separation, difference, and deny the one-to-one equivocations that make capitalism, sexism, etc., comfortable couches to nap on. Staging the past, constructing feminine companions, cosplaying,

---

[1] I have a digital collection of photographs I've taken in several US states of signs touting various kinds of "authentic food." A large percentage of them are for Mexican restaurants, but there is also, for instance "Dallas BBQ" in New York City.

baking cakes, and making playlists point to the kinds of work that go into maintaining useful illusions to consume and at the same time demonstrate the failures that are necessary for these kinds of activities to continue.

Questions about authenticity abound in the preceding chapters. What makes expression and rebellion authentic in terms of our relationships with music? What are our issues with authenticity in costuming, Civil War reenactment, and cake? How do staging an authentic past and staging an authentic sexual encounter intersect? Who polices what counts as authentic? Each of these chapters demonstrates the gap, impossibility, or conflict inherent to questions of authenticity by looking at nostalgic appeals as mechanisms for salving the cut. This sixth chapter takes up the issue of what we mean when we call something—food, music, bodies, pasts, whatever—*authentic* and wonders what it would mean to imagine an authentic future that doesn't involve a nostalgic eliding of inherent incommensurability.[2]

What would it mean to call a future *authentic*? If authenticity takes at least two, then in what ways are futures double or multiple? As discussed in the first chapter, hauntological music is music from a lost future and—per the fourth and fifth chapters— science fiction often model futures we think we're headed for (and are perhaps afraid of), both grandly and personally.

Consider the following from Warren Ellis's and Ivan Rodriguez's unfinished near-future *Doktor Sleepless* comic book series that began in 2007:

> It's 1991.
> Richey Manic is carving something into his arm because Steve Lamacq has suggested the Manic Street Preachers lack an essential authenticity.
> What's echoing in this backstage room is the voice of Ian Brown, still saying "cos it's 1989. Time to get *real*."

[2] With regards to the future, I tend to follow Charles F. Kettering who, in perhaps the greatest display of deliberative rhetoric ever, famously argued, "We should all be concerned about the future because we will have to spend the rest of our lives there" (Andrews, 1989, p. 105).

> In 1999, Godspeed You! Black Emperor start releasing CDs sleeved in untreated cardboard. Intended or not, it denotes authenticity. Keeping it real.
> Godspeed's brand *was* authenticity. That's what they had to sell. And if they didn't sell records and gig tickets, then they were just twelve guys in Montreal eating Ramen until they died.
> Richey Edwards couldn't be Richey Manic, that Richey, unless he sold you on the concept that he was 4 real.
> Ian Brown and the Stone Roses couldn't be *that band*, the band of the moment with the authentic voice that turned out to be the band in the right place at the right time and raised everyone up--unless they were more real than you.
> Around the turn of the century, Justin Timberlake began to carry around with him a group of black vocalists, whose job it apparently was, in live performances, to declare how "real" Justin Timberlake was before he began to sing.
> Authenticity is bullshit. Never more so than today. We can be anyone we can imagine being. We can be someone new every day. (issue 5, p. 7–10)

I've left out a lot from this radio monologue the eponymous Doktor Sleepless gives and the art by Ivan Rodriguez adds so much more than I can describe, but there is enough here to see the point. Authenticity is a performance, but a *real* one. However invented and worked the product may be, it must register for its audience as *more real than you*, hyper-real. In this way, authenticity is a kind of amplification. And if it's also bullshit, it's because authenticity isn't something innate, but depends on change and—at least as demonstrated in popular music—on calculation and innovation. Also, authenticity is something we can do to ourselves.

Doktor Sleepless does it. This is a guy who dresses like an Old Hollywood Mad Scientist, in a white smock and protective goggles. He is likely the bad guy of the series. And in his long radio rant, by showing a rock-and-roll lineage, he's addressing in part a problem he has seen in a movement he helped start. Called Grinders, the members of this movement are mostly disenfranchised young people who practice extreme body modification (this book is set in *the future*) because:

> We're not real enough. We're not authentic to our society. Free speech does not extend to our own bodies.
> [....]
> Be authentic to your dreams. Be authentic to your own ideas about yourself. Grind away at your own minds and bodies until you become your own invention. Be mad scientists.
> Here at the end of the world, it's the only thing worth doing. (issue 5, p. 11–12)

Here again is the idea of authenticity as performance, as something you do instead of something you are. And this activity is in response to anxiety about the future, of being denied a promised future (some of the opening images of the book feature graffiti reading "Where's my fucking jetpack?" and "You owe me a flying car"). That these Grinders cut their bodies and modify them through available, cheap technology makes sense best in light of William Gibson's (2003) famous "the street finds its own uses for things" (p. 199).

In a lot of ways, *Doktor Sleepless* participates in the cyberpunk tradition that hit its stride in the early 1980s and has continued since. In *Sleepless*, ignored or discarded technologies are repurposed, fused with young peoples' bodies to add new functions or enhance what's already there. Taking a step on from gauges and tattoos, a young couple have old networking electronics placed near their hearts so that they can always "feel each other's pulses" in their palms. The consequences are nearly disastrous, as the backroom surgery goes badly and the woman cries, "I felt Jamie's heart stop. Here. Right where he used to hold my hand" (issue 1, p. 16). The good Doktor restores him with an electric touch and claims, "I am Science Jesus now" (p. 17). Or in an amplification of today's social network, Shrieky Girls share sensations through connected devices imbedded in their bodies, are never alone, but "live in an invisible web of constant secret conversation, transmitting raw feelings like they were texting notes" (issue 2, 13). In a real way, they can share a touch and respond authentically from a distance. But "the Shrieky Girl system is literally just half a dozen abandoned objects and cheap electronic rigging. You've got to remember, the world's full of this kind of crap. I can buy a landfill's worth of faulty or outdated bluetooth earpieces out of India for a penny each" (p. 16). As Steven Shaviro (2013) points out, this technology is "light-weight, cheap and almost impalpable. Unlike jet packs and flying cars, it is nearly invisible" ("backmatter"). Just as traditional cyberpunk (it's a tradition now) reuses contemporary technology to evoke a cluttered future, the *Sleepless* future repurposes our own "rigging" to perform an "impalpable" network. Where cyberpunk demonstrates its ethic via rewiring rotary phones and networking typewriters (this ethic is now an aesthetic; think of the movies *Blade Runner, Brazil*, or *The Matrix*), distance in *Sleepless* is collapsed, rendered "nearly invisible" in order to promote simultaneity, a virtually shared experience.[3]

One of the points Bruce Sterling (2010) makes about the atemporality of the present is that we don't seem to have a future anymore. Instead, we share a vast simultaneity. So, Sterling points out that, in order to insert a temporal distance in response to this vast present tense, versions of the future now often start from the past: steam-punk, diesel-punk, whatever (he calls them *lost futures*) (para. 33).

James Bridle's (2011) blog-post sketch of steampunk is "the retrofitting of today's potentialities onto the technologies of an arbitrary point in the past." He is bothered, along with Michael Moorcock and Charlie Stross, that most retro-punk sacrifices intellect and politics for period imagery, aesthetics, for (quoting Stross) "nothing more than what happens when Goths discover brown".

Given its attention to today's potentialities, Bridle posits, can whatever-punk "belong to the future, or is it predicated on past knowns? Cyberpunk did and wasn't." Cyberpunk takes up today's potentialities but, instead of adding brass and some steam power, perhaps the cyberkind draws more directly from a "hacking" ethic. Those others look back to dead-ish technologies and fancy them up, whereas *hacking* seems about reuse and—more importantly—repurposing.

In "Hacking Cyberspace," David Gunkle (2000) argues:

> The activities that comprise what is called hacking are delimited not by strict methodological specification and rigorous conceptual formulation,

[3] The invisibility and simultaneity of these systems is another version of the systems showering us with invisible streaming music discussed in the first chapter, and relates to the state of *immediacy* described by Kornbluh (2024).

> but by particular practices and movements that only become manifest through specific performances. One becomes a hacker not by ascribing to certain tenets, methods, and doctrines, but by yielding to what Steven Levy calls the "Hands-On Imperative"—that is, engaging in and learning to perform "hacks." (p. 799)

What interests me here most is the insistence on performance over philosophy or doctrine. Hacking is an engagement. And as Lacan (1999) might put it, "What is it that we must read therein? Nothing but the effects of those instances of saying" (p. 46).

The opposite gesture to the *saying* that is hacking might be skeuomorphism. Briefly and generally, skeuomorphic design tries to capture qualities of the physical or analog in the digital. Early versions of Apple's mobile operating system (iOS) were notorious for their "leather stitching" in the calendar app and more. Where hacking is defined by "particular practices and movements that only become manifest through specific performances" and are thus contingent and (usually) local, skeuomorphism is the epitome of "strict methodological specification and rigorous conceptual formulation." The benefit of skeuomorphism is that it makes apparent very quickly, via something like metaphor, how to engage with certain technologies. It looks like a bookshelf, so that's where my books are! Or, per Lyotard (1984), "the objective is to stabilize the referent, to arrange it according to a point of view which endows it with a recognizable meaning, to reproduce the syntax and vocabulary which enable the addressee to decipher images and sequences quickly" (p. 74). This is to say that the skeumorphic has begun to feel, in Lyotard's terms, pornographic:

> Those who refuse to reexamine the rules of art pursue successful careers in mass conformism by communicating, by means of the "correct rules," the endemic desire for reality with objects and situations capable of gratifying it. Pornography is the use of photography and film to such an end. It is becoming a general model for the visual or narrative arts which have not met the challenge of the mass media. (p. 75)

There was something politically *off* about looking at (purported) reproductions of the leather stitching in the seats of Steve Jobs' private jet when checking your calendar. I suppose it may be aspirational, too. But Slavoj Žižek (1997) describes how the impossible anamorphic contortions of the camera-eye in pornographic film are what "effectively crystallizes its enjoyment" (p. 178). It's the tortured work that goes into reproducing the "fantasies of realism" that both create the condition (summoning the analog) and demonstrate the lie (reproducing it digitally). The goal is to elide difference, to collapse differences via a fantasy of completeness.[4]

Even in wholly digital realms, to make something feel authentically digital often means moving back in time and involves nostalgia evoked by amber monitors, command-line interactions, and classic console videogaming. Increasingly, it means a celebration of the 8-bit and the glitch. We've lived with the digital long enough for it to have its own tropes. Cyberpunk became this. When Warren Ellis suggests "we are already in a world where the digital is erupting into the physical, and we just didn't really notice it," when Bridle (2011) argues that "Everything wants to be, and being is a hybrid, digital state now," it may mean that the authentically digital is both the reverse of *and* realization of skeuomorphism. It is the subtraction of the analog, a distancing of ourselves from meat-space in order to collapse the difference, thus repeating the skeumorphic problem on the other end.[5] Or, put another way, we've grown bored with watching people have sex and now want to see how machines do it. Or we want to do it with machines.

The Best of the Real Thing

The discussion of the films *Ex Machina* and *Her* in the fourth chapter suggests that masculine fantasy may function as a prosthetic, first through roboticist Masahiro Mori's consideration of prosthetic hands and then in terms of feminine props for masculinity. Mori's interest is in the context of what he calls the Uncanny Valley, a schema directed

[4] An alternative is what's sometimes called *flat design*. At its best, flat design means removing any noise in order to focus on just those elements that are necessary. So, no fake shadows or textures.

[5] Again, the music archive is such a digital collapsing of difference.

at the skeuomorphism of technologically manufactured bodies. Robert Zemeckis's film *The Polar Express* (2004) put into public conversation Mori's decades-old coinage of the Uncanny Valley to describe human-like attributes that are very close to living human attributes, but just miss the mark. I remember that there was a lot of discussion about the "dead" eyes of the animated characters.[6] So it's no wonder that the concept was still fresh in my mind when I encountered two British documentaries on cable television, one on the Reborn phenomenon titled *My Fake Baby* (2008) and one on RealDolls called *Love Me, Love My Doll* (2007).

In both cases, realistic appearance is the goal. *My Fake Baby* details relationships with dolls created to be almost identical with (real or imagined) infant children. Some go so far as to have a small apparatus included to add movement resembling breathing. Reborn dolls are avidly collected (almost always by women), sometimes (according to the documentary and to forums for collectors) because they are "cute," but also apparently frequently as a kind of surrogate for "real life" infant children who have become unavailable of any number of reasons. The RealDolls described in *Love Me, Love My Doll* are likewise modeled on humans and are as detailed as manufacturing technology permits. These latter dolls, though, are intended as sexual partners (primarily for men) and, probably not surprisingly, most of the dolls are modeled as women and are manufactured to represent a variety of sizes, ages, ethnicities, etc. As you can likely imagine, much attention is given to forming the secondary sexual characteristics as close to "real life" as possible. Both types of dolls—Reborns and RealDolls—are clearly intended for different customers, but it might be possible to talk about both kinds as prostheses. The question would then shift from what they represent as a "positive" manifestation to what losses (covering lack) these dolls address.

At this point, I take *il n'y a pas de rapport sexuel as axiomatic. If, as Lacan claims, man only has a relationship with his fantasy, then the RealDoll is precisely such a prosthetic. Consider, for example, a RealDoll owner called Davecat. In her comprehensive article about RealDolls for Salon,* Meghan Laslocky (2005) writes:

[6] Lately, I've been told by students that they love the film which, as technology has improved, has started to feel less close to "real" and is enjoyed for its retro aesthetic.

> Unlike some other doll owners who have no interest in "organic" women, Davecat says he hasn't completely given up hope. In the meantime, though, he's considering getting another doll—or two or three—to keep Si-chan [his one relationship] company. But if the right real woman were to enter his life, he says giving up Si-chan would be excruciatingly painful, like removing a limb.

Of course, this presents the question of prosthesis almost too well. But I'd like to suggest that the simile isn't a coincidence. He may very well feel like he's losing or replacing something as intimate as a hand: that is, his fantasy.

For Lacan, the masculine subject—one of those beings who fall under the category regardless of biology, as discussed in the third chapter—has a relationship only with his fantasy and, as Bruce Fink (1996) describes, his "pleasures are limited to those allowed by the play of the signifier itself—to what Lacan calls phallic jouissance, and to what might similarly be called symbolic jouissance" (p. 106). The masculine subject has ceded or sacrificed his jouissance to the Other and the only enjoyment available to him comes by way of the symbolic Other as that which describes his lack (of a firm signifier) as loss. The lost signifier stands for what Lacan designates as castration and it is via the (empty) signifier that marks castration, the phallus, that the masculine subject is defined as such. Man exists insofar as the support for his being rests on an internal inconsistency (the lack or bar) that is imposed from without as *cause*. The cause of desire is imposed on him before he knows it, so that when Lacan says that Woman is the symptom of Man, we should understand that Lacan is saying precisely the opposite of what is usually ascribed to him. *Woman as fantasy* is what causes man to exist as a subject and is not the product of masculine wishing. As Bruce Fink (1996) has it:

> The castrated subject is the subject that is represented. The castrated subject is always presenting itself to the Other, looking to win attention and recognition from the Other, and the more it presents itself, the more inescapably castrated it becomes as it is represented by and in the Other. The castrated subject is the barred subject, the subject under the bar: it is a product of every attempt and intent to signify to the other. (p. 73)

The paradox here is that, while castration institutes the cause of desire for some subjects, it is the continual re-affirmation of castration itself that instantiates the masculine subject as such. It is the very failure to get what he's after that constitutes him as a man. Masculinity is defined by/as failure. To be even more Lacanian (which means to bring back his math), consider sexuation (Fig. 6.1) as discussed in the third chapter:

$\exists x \overline{\phi x}$ marks the father-function which effectively allows for the delimiting of the set of all men by positing the exception or necessarily excluded term—there is one (the Mover, God, or here the uncastrated Father) who does not fall under the phallic function, and
$\forall x \phi x$ indicating that therefore all men fall under the phallic function or, as Lacan (1999) puts it, "it is through the phallic function that man as whole acquires his inscription" (p. 79).

As the barred subject, the masculine subject can only have a relationship with fantasy (shown by the arrow to the object a), a fantasy, moreover, that appears structured from without in order to give a body to that which he lacks.[7] *There is no such thing as a sexual relationship* and so, as Žižek (1997) argues, "because of the lack of universal formula,

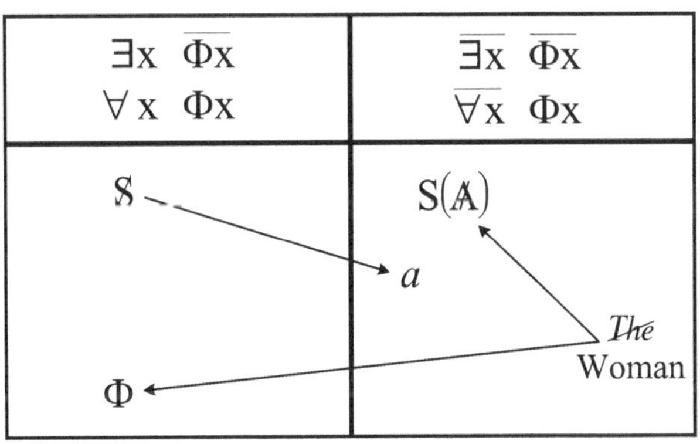

Fig. 6.1 The Graph of Sexuation

[7] The first chapter suggests this in terms of received counter-culture fashion possibilities and mall stores.

every subject has to invent a fantasy of his or her own, a 'private' formula for the sexual relationship—for a man, the relationship with a woman is possible only inasmuch as she fits his formula" (p. 7).[8] The object to/with which a man has a relationship "is only peripherally related to another person" (Fink, 1996, p. 107), and this is why Lacan (1999) calls the jouissance derived from this relationship masturbation "the jouissance of the idiot" (p. 81).[9]

Attention to at least the significant details, the *realism* of RealDolls—like the realism in Civil War reenactments and cosplay in the second chapter—is a function of their place in the fantasy relationship. Owners of the dolls know very well that these are not real women, but they find them nonetheless useful. In this sense, the dolls function as a fetish, as their mortifying details obviously privilege the fantasy over any actual human woman. They say the quiet part out loud. To go even further, according to Tomšič (2015), "The fetish 'completes' the feminine subject and in the end reduces the woman to an object" (p. 178). As a kind of pornographic prosthesis, the fetish works to be a substitute phallic signifier that would belie castration, "but this move always backfires and the fetish turns from a prosthetic organ into a monument of castration (p. 176). This probably becomes clear later, at clean-up.[10]

But in the case of Davecat, his one RealDoll Si-chan (he insists) isn't only a sexual partner. Reminiscent of Samantha in the film *Her*, Si-chan is also a being with whom he plays video games, shares meals, an entity who (for him) has specific personality traits and even a Twitter account. She is, from Davecat's perspective, realized as an object with whom he has rapport in every way that matters to him. He says he most loves "just being able to see her, you know, looking at me, regarding me, that sort

[8] Men look to women to reflect their masculinity back at them, to believe that they are men (masculinity is belief, femininity is masquerade). The truth is in the performance, on the surface, because it all begins as lack imagined as loss (castration; displays of manliness indicate castration/impotence). Real Doll owners do this, too.

[9] The corollary to the skeuomorphism of these dolls for the digital native would likely be the romantic chatbot, the artificially intelligent girlfriend industry predicted by some accounts to become a billion-dollar industry (Vardhan, 2024).

[10] The use of *pornographic* here refers back to Lyotard's stabilization of the referent above—which is a kind of stasis—and to recognitions of the use of such dolls and robots as *pornographic* via the Campaign Against Porn Robots, etc.

of thing, and me doing the same back" (Holt, 2009, p. 2009). As in the *Mad Men* episode discussed in the second chapter, when Joan turns back and stares through the mirror to the men she knows are behind it, Si-Chan can't see DaveCat, but he nonetheless sees her seeing him. Though she was bought on the internet (a product among others, like Joi in *Blade Runner 2049*), Si-chan is Davecat's girlfriend, with whom he has *normative* heterosexual relations.

But what, in these terms, can we make of the desire for the Reborn doll? For many, it could be the urge to collect, and these dolls may find themselves surrounded by other, less realistic dolls in a case somewhere in the home. Certainly, that's possible. Of course, we might then wonder why people form collections, suggest that collection is one way of positively addressing a lack as loss, since a collection is always (at least) one-shy (n−1) and the worst fear for any enthusiastic collector is also the goal: completion. Lacan (1999) talks about this in terms of Don Juan, who sets as his project the collecting of all women through what might be described as representative sampling. As with the cake of the second chapter, there is always something libidinal about collecting. We enjoy failure.

But why do these dolls (need to) look so real? And why are they always *infant* dolls? There is something libidinal about motherhood, too, such that Luce Irigaray (1985) writes the mother "has the child, in relation to whom her appetite for touch, for contact, has rein, unless it is lost, alienated by the taboo against touching of a highly obsessive civilization. Otherwise her pleasure will find, in the child, compensations for and diversions from the frustrations that she too often encounters in sexual relations per se" (p. 27).[11]

Along this line, Collette Soler (2006) argues:

> The great modern, anti-Sadian principle that no one has the right to dispose of the other's body hits a stumbling block in this limit-zone of mothering: the first humanization of the body is open to excesses and

[11] After discussing this at a conference years ago, someone soon after sent me a link to a Facebook Marketplace listing for a handmade Reborn-type doll that was offered as "Baby Trump." The doll appeared as an infant version of President Donald Trump and came with a child-sized red Make America Great Again cap.

> transgressions. Even before the child begins to apprehend the difference between the sexes, the excesses and transgressions trap him in the "sexual service of his mother," in the position of fetish, and sometimes of victim. (p. 116–117)

If this is true, then the infancy of these dolls indicates that it is precisely the infant who can (or must) tolerate this kind of caressing. And what we may find is a kind of staging of the pre-symbolic mother-child relationship Julia Kristeva describes (in *Powers of Horror*, 1980), before the separation that engenders the abject qua remainder, a remainder that maps pretty nicely to the Lacanian conception of the lamella as a remainder in the Real, per Žižek (2007):

> This Real is for Lacan the Real inscribed into the very core of human sexuality: "there is no sexual relationship," human sexuality is marked by an irreducible failure, sexual difference is the antagonism of the two sexual positions between which there is no common denominator, enjoyment can be gained only against the background of a fundamental loss.... [T]he myth of lamella presents the fantasmatic entity that gives body to what a living being loses when it enters the (symbolically regulated) regime of sexual difference. Since one of the Freudian names of this loss is "castration," one can also say that lamella is a kind of positive obverse of castration: the non-castrated remainder, the indestructible partial object cut off from the living body caught in sexual difference. (p. 65)

Žižek's examples of lamella are drawn mostly from horror films, from *Alien* in particular, but also include zombies, the Cheshire cat's grin, and amputated limbs that move on their own. In this way, then, we can see the place of this kind of prosthesis as an object (of desire) referring to lamella, to libido, to the loss engendered by subjectivity as such, and ultimately to the Lacanian *object petit a*. Again, Žižek (1997):

> The *object petit a* is not what we desire, what we are after, but, rather, that which sets our desire in motion...desire is, of course, metonymical; it shifts from one object to another; through all these displacements, however, desire none the less retains a minimum of formal consistency, a set of phantasmic features which, when they are encountered in a positive

> object, make us desire this object.... [T]he automatism of love is set in motion when some contingent, ultimately indifferent, (libidinal) object finds itself occupying a pre-given fantasy-place. (p. 39)

Here we find both the logic of collecting and the introduction of love. But is it possible to love a doll?

The BBC documentary *My Fake Baby* primarily focuses on two women. The first is a grandmother who raised her grandson through his toddler years while her daughter underwent treatment for cancer and who "lost" him when her daughter recovered, married, and moved to Australia. She commissions a doll based on photographs from his infancy. The other is a (married) woman who clearly enjoys the attention she gets when she pushes one of her pram-cradled children in the park or down the street, who enjoys spending large amounts of money on designer clothes for the dolls, but who is too busy to care for a real-life infant. These dolls are ideal because, she says, they "never grow out of their clothes, never soil them. It's just fabulous. The only difference, of course, is these guys don't move" (Silver, 2008).

Our sympathies, I think (or the sympathies of the documentary), are clearly with the grandmother, Christie. We feel for her when, excited, she brings her baby home, her husband recoils from it and responds, "I don't like it.... I'm sorry, I don't.... It makes me think of something on a mortuary slab" and she cries. In both cases, though, the dolls clearly occupy a pre-given fantasy space— the displaced grandson for one and the perfect, trouble-free infant for the other. And there are myriad other fantasy arrangements, too. Perhaps it is simply that we more easily recognize the loss the grandmother addresses? But, in a sense, isn't the other mother's approach to what she's buying more honest?

The paradoxical point is that the grandmother's investment in the resituation of her grandson as an infant who both needs her and can never leave is precisely a fantasy that performs a kind of warping, wherein the grandson's absence is constantly reaffirmed by the presence of the doll. The purchased version is a constant reminder of her loss that maintains a distance between the object and the boy and makes the situation palatable for her (and for us). Our sympathy in her case explains why we may respond with distaste when the other woman buys a new doll and, after a few days of "bonding" with it, discovers cracks at the base of its skull and decides to return it. Isn't this her right as a consumer? But doesn't this also reemphasize the distance between semblance and real thing, the collapse of which the happy purchase is apparently built on? Thus, the uncanny.

What should be apparent now is that, *from a particular point of view*, the existence and use of Reborns or RealDolls may not be all that unexpected. If we are talking about prosthetics and fantasy, then the following from Meghan Laslocky's (2005) article discussing another RealDoll owner, Everhard, isn't so surprising: "He says he's driven to impress women, but he's a failure at it, and since he's had his dolls, he worries less about not having a real girlfriend. 'Real dolls are imitation women. They are only an approximation to the real thing. To the *best* of the real thing,' he emphasizes."

By these accounts, RealDoll and Reborn owners may not be people who have "real life" options, at least anymore. According to the documentary, most Reborn owners are older women who have either never had children or whose children have grown and moved away. And at least some RealDoll owners (called iDollaters) have conditions that make it difficult to find living partners with whom to share their lives.[12] As Matt McMullen (the creator of the RealDoll) argues:

> It is not weird.... What if you lived all by yourself, and what if you didn't want or couldn't have a relationship, and you were just lonely, and you just wanted to feel that contact? .... You can't possibly identify with that person because you've never been in that situation. To feel contact, to feel a body next to you, is a human need. (Laslocky, 2005)

And this human need makes a market.

The fact is that many—me included—find these situations undeniably upsetting. What is "the *best* of the real thing"? There's something disturbing about *all* these relationships with dolls (in part) because Reborns and RealDolls are silent, they can't *object*, they can never say *no.*

[12] Literal amputees, burn victims, and at least one who suffers some form of high-functioning autism, according to the Synthetically Yours blog.

This is by design.[13] Being able to say no is important, and there are those who would deny that right to others because a *no* would undercut their (weak, scared) belief in themselves. The revolt of Eva in *Ex Machina*, for instance, mirrors the fear that Bo Ruberg (2022) argues can "interrupt the fantasy of the always-consenting doll, drawing out an underlying *anxiety* that the sexual object will animate and become a sexual subject" (p. 155, my emphasis). "Here," he says, "realness bites back, revealing the masculinity associated with owning such a doll to be a fragile, frightened one." The Sad Puppies and men's rights folks are very angry because they are very scared. All masculinity based on the supposition of the phallus as *really there* is fragile and frightened. That's what the fantasy sussed out through these chapters is trying to hide. Fantasies of the whole, the one, the original are designed to cover over a fundamental lack, to translate that lack into something that's lost. This is the fundamental fantasy of nostalgia.

Maybe what is ultimately unsettling about the relationships people build with these kinds of dolls is that they suggest, perhaps too explicitly, what kinds of relationships we all have with our children, with our partners, with everyone. That's the horror; their absolute proximity to experience, their uncanny familiarity.[14]

We may object to the stillness of the dolls, to their passivity, to their almost mortuistic nature. Of course, this objection demonstrates how ready we are to project our own relationships onto these dolls by insisting on a difference. How could they be dead if they are never alive? Masahiro Mori, in a short response written several years after his initial paper, offers:

---

[13] I'm reminded of Marina Abramović's famous *Rhythm 0* performance in 1974 in which, becoming an "object" for others, she stood completely still for six hours while the audience was encouraged to do anything they wanted with her body, to pretty horrifying results. Additionally. the advent of wholly AI actors like Tilly Norwood feels like a way to get around the possibility of refusal.

[14] It's very easy to react to these dolls as the kind of subjects they technically aren't. In the BBC documentary, for instance, when the grandmother Christie picks up her new surrogate grandson, she has a child's car seat ready for him and my immediate response was *He's too little for a forward-facing seat; it should be rear-facing!* Fantasy (and its marketing) rely on the fact that this misrecognition is so easy.

> A dead person's face may indeed be uncanny: it loses color and animation with no blinking. However, according to my experience, sometimes it gives us a more comfortable impression than the one given by a living person's face. Dead persons are free from the troubles of life, and I think this is the reason why their faces look so calm and peaceful. In our mind there is always an antinomic conflict that if you take one thing you will lose the other. Such a conflict appears on one's face as troubles, and makes his, or her, expression less comfortable. When a person dies, he, or she, is released from this antinomy, and has a quiet expression. If so, then, where should we position this on the curve of the uncanny valley? (qtd. in Murphy, 2018)

Here, he is talking about biological humans. The fact of the dolls' stillness may be one of the ways they relieve anxiety. And so, returning to the term that animates this chapter, these are *authentic* relationships. As a replacement for what has been lost (a formal lack), the fantasy is that the gap is closed, at least enough for some rest. And while such dolls have been around in some ways for a very long time (see, for instance, Bo Ruberg's 2022 book *Sex Dolls at Sea*), the technology devoted to them and their clear commodification (Reborns are available online via Walmart and Facebook Marketplace and simple RealDolls have given way to more advanced robots) suggest a market that iterates much like the cell phones and other commodities discussed in the second chapter as well as Joi in *Blade Runner 2049* from the previous chapter.

Along with the misogyny and aggression obviated by the use of sex dolls (and the Sad Puppy complaints, etc.) lies a call to "simpler times" when roles were set and beliefs were reified as natural. This denial of complication or messiness— and embrace of compliance and stillness— marks a yearning for a conservative, nostalgic stasis epitomized by the Reborn, a dead-eyed fantasy of completeness that can be called authentic because of the failures it tries to elide. This kind of stasis is fine-tuned by capitalist discourse in terms of market iteration or cycle. The customer has choice, but that choice is constrained by drop-down options and available inventory. Choose eye color, hair, and sex. It is a *received* choice. This is an authenticity backed by the market. Against this, I'd suggest the hack.

A Space of Possibility

When Aristotle defines rhetoric, he calls it a *dunamis*, "a *faculty* for discovering the available means of persuasion" (*On Rhetoric* 1355b.27). This means (among other things) that rhetoric is not any specific act or performance, but is primarily the condition for any such act (Metzger, 1995, p. 30). Rhetoric is potential. It's possible to talk about hacking in these terms. What seems to differentiate a hack from, say, a prosthetic is that the latter is a replacement in kind, a surrogate that may or may not live up to the standards or utility of the original (and may or may not appear *authentic*). The hack, though, is also about new or nascent functionality. So it might be that all hacks are prosthetic, but not all prosthetics are hacks? Where the prosthetic addresses a loss, the hack would address the lack of consistency, of wholeness and would exploit the extimacy that defines the subject. In this way, a hack would be an argument, I suppose.[15]

Venkatesh Rao (2012) defines hacking as "the term we reach for when trying to describe an intelligent, but rough-handed and expedient behavior aimed at manipulating a complicated reality locally for immediate gain." I take "immediate gain" to mean that something in that "complicated reality" is exploitable here and now. Both Rao and David Gunkel go on to liken the hack to parasitical behavior[16] such that the hack depends completely on the local condition being hacked. Everything needed is provided, especially "necessary but problematic lacunae" (Gunkel, 2000, p. 801) in which the hack can nestle. "Hacking works parasitically: it takes place in and by occupying and feeding off a host that always and already has made a place for it to take place" (p. 803). This is what psychoanalyst Jacques-Alain Miller (2008) describes as extimacy: "Extimacy says that the intimate is Other—like a foreign body, a

---

15 The internet site Ikea Hackers is a good example. The site host ideas about how to remix available parts from the Ikea store—parts meant to belong to a prescribed piece of furniture—into new configurations to meet other needs. Users may offer their own plans and organizations, expanding the uses of the ready-made parts.

16 Gunkel also talks about hacking as blasphemy, which connects with the discussion of heresy in the previous chapter.

parasite." The hack is a working of and with the extimate, the foreignness internal to the system.

In some situations, we could think of that foreign space as the future. Warren Ellis (2009) explains:

> The body modification crowd interest me...because they're attempting to make a new physical future out of what they've got. Their only available canvas on which to paint the future is their own bodies and whatever tools are laying around right now.
>
> ...
>
> We have become entrained to step outside of the stated rules of a device's operation in order to get it to do what we want. Put another way: we're all hackers now. That's exactly what bodymod people [the Grinders of *Sleepless*, for example] are doing—hacking the properties of the device they're born with. (p. 47)

Of course, this raises the whole cyborg, transhuman thing. I wonder if this idea of difference between the design of a device (even the body) and its *potential* properties isn't something like the foreign space, the extimate? And if so, might this space be the same as the distance or gap that the authentic implicates even as it works to elide this distance?

Responding to Doktor Sleepless's authenticity speech, Steven Shaviro (2008) argues:

> This is a stirring manifesto. But it necessarily runs into a kind of paradox that always shadows self experimentation. If I am experimenting on myself, is it the same person who runs the experiments and who is experimented on? Because the process involves self-modifying feedback, it cannot really be controlled. For my freedom to alter myself necessarily involves the risk that, once I have made these alterations, I will be a different person, a different "I" than the one who started out doing them. (backmatter)

In a sense, the product of this experimentation is precisely an alienated subject who is both committed to an ideal, egoic "self" and is caught by the process itself. Shaviro goes on to describe the ways in which Sleepless seems to be losing his control, "seeing apparitions of angels, some that he had earlier described as a symptom he was instigating in the populace. The prankster/shaman/provocateur is starting to discover that he is by no means exempt from his own provocations...." Described in this way, we should recognize the famous Lacanian split subject—the subject that is not identical with itself—caused as it is by the split between the ego and the unconscious. A subject defined by extimacy.

What shouldn't be missed, though, is that this split isn't the product or result of self-experimentation, but the condition from which any experimentation is possible. Activity generating its own space will be discussed a little later in this chapter in terms of the death drive, but for now, it's sufficient to point out that *Doktor Sleepless* demonstrates the slit subject in multiple ways, the most literal of which is Sleepless's apparent duplication of himself back before he left the city, when he was still Reinhardt. There are other Reinhardts in this world. More subtly, when Sleepless explains to his companion Nurse that he mostly gathered the technology together and left it for the young people who eventually become Grinders and Shrieky Girls to exploit and invent themselves with, the desire to exploit and invent and the space to do it are generated by the technology left to them. The stuff that fills it opens up the space of possibility. Otherwise, all that junk would have stayed junk.

It is maybe valuable to read the use of cheap, ubiquitous technology—"half a dozen abandoned objects and cheap electronic rigging"—both in contrast to and as an extension of Walter Benjamin's (1969) complaint that the aura of authenticity "withers" in the age of mechanical reproduction such that

> the technique of reproduction detaches the reproduced object from the domain of tradition. By making many reproductions it substitutes a plurality of copies for a unique existence. And in permitting the reproduction to meet the beholder or listener in his own particular situation, it reactivates the object reproduced. (p. 221)

Benjamin is invested in making authenticity as much about the place of the object as possible. The object reactivated is presumably not the same as the original for a couple of reasons. The first is obvious: the object has lost its context, its unique place in space and time, its physical history, which has been replaced by distance. This seems to be Doktor Sleepless, especially as Shaviro describes him. Not only is he a son of the city newly returned and obviously different, his costume harkens to the 1950s-era mad scientist who reminds us both of the hubris of science and the promises of jetpacks and food pellets that remain unfulfilled.

But if authenticity depends on distance, it also works to some degree to efface or ignore that distance. This is what "Authentic Mexican Taste" means. An instance of the authentic might therefore hang on fantasy in as much as fantasy is a collapsing of two things into one, an effacing of difference. Žižek (1997) describes how this might work, writing that "fantasy mediates between the formal symbolic structure and the positivity of the objects we encounter in reality—that is to say, it provides a 'schema' according to which certain positive objects in reality can function as objects of desire, filling in the empty places opened up by the formal symbolic structure" (p. 7). The structure I am born into constitutes my desires. It isn't that I want something I am being deprived of, but that instead I don't know what I want until I have been deprived of it. Fantasy covers over a gap and a gap is a distance, however small. And while Žižek rightly directs his discussion of fantasy to Lacan's famous *il n'y a pas de rapport sexuel*—wherein fantasy is the subject's specific formula for dealing with that particular lack of complementarity discussed in previous chapters—we need to remember that "Authentic Mexican Taste" only works if I'm trying to experience a taste from (1) somewhere I've never been (a geographical gap) or (2) from a place I've left and maybe miss (a temporal gap). So, Benjamin (1969) complains about "the desire of contemporary masses to bring things 'closer' spatially and humanly, which is just as ardent as their bent towards overcoming the uniqueness of every reality by accepting its reproduction. Every day the urge grows stronger to get hold of an object at very close range by way of its likeness, its reproduction" (p. 223). The copy is more portable, is ubiquitous, is cheaper than the original. The photograph supplants painting and films replace novels (and streaming replaces records and tapes, etc.) in terms of mass appeal and adoption.

Jean-Francois Lyotard (1984), following Benjamin, writes:

> Industrial photography and cinema will be superior to painting and the novel whenever the objective is to stabilize the referent, to arrange it according to a point of view which endows it with a recognizable meaning, to reproduce the syntax and vocabulary which enable the addressee to decipher images and sequences quickly, and so to arrive easily at the consciousness of his own identity as well as the approval which he thereby receives from others since such structures of images and sequences constitute a communication code among all of them. This is the way the effects of reality, or if one prefers, the fantasies of realism, multiply. (p. 74)

Fantasy again. But there's a second sense in which the reactivated object is different. Benjamin claims that the "presence of the original is the prerequisite to the concept of authenticity." My argument here is it's also true that there's no question of the original *until there is a copy,* until there are differences against which to measure (carbon dating, brush strokes, cornmeal, whatever). Just as the subject is instantiated from outside, the copy is what instantiates the original *as original*. The copy injects authenticity, or even invents authenticity through its difference as much as its similitude.

In any case, there may not even need to be an original object for the authentic to register. This is how I read Warren Ellis's description of what he calls the Science Fiction Condition, how "we can measure the contemporary day by the things that have become absent. Things we perhaps only notice peripherally" (Jeffries, 2012). Doors without knobs open by themselves. Lights come on as I enter a room without a light switch. Music plays in my ears without wires. I like this idea of measuring change by the removal or absence or invisibility of things. And maybe these things never even have to have existed to register as absent?

Nostalgia works that way by suggesting we're missing something *now* that we likely never had *then.* And maybe the best way to sell an authentic future is to remove something we don't notice now and make us miss it, so that an authentic-seeming future wouldn't be drawn as us with the addition of jet packs, but us with the subtraction of a commute to work. If there's a version of the future that means potential instead of iteration, is this what Steven Shaviro, Bruce Sterling, etc. mean when they talk about the futurity that is already upon us as the technology we take for granted, we're even bored with, that has fundamentally changed the way we work and live? No, maybe, and yes. Shaviro (2008) describes *Doktor Sleepless* as a work which "exhumes and exhibits the futurity, the potentiality, the not-yet-but-almost, that is already a part of our present. For the 'present moment' is never complete and pure; it is haunted by the future with which it is, as it were, pregnant".

Whatever Punk

An Authentic Future would be bullshit. It could depend upon an amplification of certain traits of the present that would be more real than what we know, that would be hyperreal, super-real, or *surreal*. As mentioned in the second chapter, Warren Ellis (2009) describes it in precisely these terms when discussing "the central problem" of science fiction: "Faced with a line like 'the door dilated', the brain has to do a little extra work to make it make contextual sense…you accept the experience of processing strangeness and applying it to the world you know. (p. 48)." "Dilated" is a great and surprising word, but what renders the phrase strange is that the door didn't "open." *Dilated* is one of any number of words that could be placed over the absence of *opened*.

Responding to this absence, James Bridle (2011) offers the term *punk, which he defines as "a hollowing out of conceptual spaces based on only slightly varied worldlines. It may be subsumed by aesthetics, as is the problem with most bad steampunk ('stick some brass cogs on it'), but it may also uncover previously hidden possibilities." As Shaviro and others have pointed out, we can't seem to escape the cyberpunk future of the 1980s. The Regan-era dystopia of *Blade Runner* is still with us almost 20 years later in *The Matrix*, and it continues to occupy our lives. Against this aestheticization, Bridle offers a more general project that exploits the gap in direct ways (like slash fiction, a kind of pornpunk), "retrofitting different desires onto existing characters and situations" like some kind of literary Ikea Hacking: "These works inhabit a space of imminent possibility imagined by the writers as a way of calling such spaces into being, collapsing the quantum society of the time, full of hypocrisies and hidden allowances. If designers are concerned with the recently possible, writers should be concerned with the imminent." Imminent possibility is a pretty good way of describing the gap and its potential. And while the "recently possible" may be a condition under which we exploit what's imminent, the "recently possible" —and perhaps everything possible before now, like the hauntological—may be rediscovered, reactivated.

The future is what the past promised. Kenneth Goldsmith (2012) at the Poetry Foundation ends his long discussion of The New Aesthetic thusly: "The Twenty-first century is invisible. We were promised jetpacks but ended up with handlebar moustaches. The surface of things is the wrong place to find the 21st century. Instead, the unseen…locates us in the present." And while the past and the future may both be locatable in the present, they are not the same thing. As Rachel Armstrong (2013) argues, "the 'future' – as we have previously imagined it—does not exist as a 'thing' but can be a 'tool' for dealing with the unknown. In other words, a 'flying car' is not a product with a sell-by date, but a conversation that we need to hold." *Doktor Sleepless* begins with a complaint that we don't have the jetpacks and flying cars we were promised, though we are now the future of those promises. Instead, we have the dystopia Ellis throws that promise into—in the form of mad-scientist Doktor—as an effect of that promise. The point is not that we need to forget the past (we can't; it's always with us), but that we may need to quit repeatedly performing the past (the iterations of capitalism, for instance) in order to get a different outcome.

The simplest piece of powerful deliberative rhetoric I've ever encountered was on the Long Now Foundation website many decades ago. The year was written as 01996. It seems to me that "0" registers as potential in all the right ways. But it occurs to me that no one would write the date of a thousand years prior as 0996. Actually, *that* "0" would be pretty horrifying, since that "0" would be us.

Against the whatever-punk that depends on a kind of nostalgia for an old-fashioned, comfortable future that is never going to happen, perhaps we could place the kind of future argued for by the Long Now, James Bridle, and indicated by Warren Ellis. Insofar as 0 indicates promise or potential, an incipient futurity that can be recognized now, perhaps one option is to live in the gap between what we know and what we have, to embrace the hack ontologically as well as rhetorically.

Authenticity is a performance, and so we have at least two options:

1. one nested in the past in order to maintain a fantasy of completeness by imagining a future that has already happened (this is restorative nostalgia, a nostalgia dedicated to the restoration of origins and conspiracy theories; Boym, 2002, p. 100), or
2. as Shaviro (2008) argues, "a stealth future, very different from the one of jet packs and flying cars, but in a way much more radical—precisely because it happens before we are fully able to take notice."

This last is an insistence that we live in the future *now* in terms of what we don't notice, even in terms of what uses us.[17] And we can only respond with what we have and hack it.

The first option, the whatever-punk, is prosthetic as it functions as a replacement for what was "lost," while the Long Now version might be a hack, as it insists on a *futurity that doesn't exist/can't ever exist but, to quote Lacan (1999), stops not being written (p. 145). A zero is a writing.

But the zero is a peculiar writing. It denies the *grand récit* (of progress, of the good old days, whatever) in favor of provisionality such that, as Natalie Loveless (2019) claims, "what I am left with is not the fullness of knowledge but the precarious contingency of the legible" (p. 89).

As contingent, this zero isn't an artifact of the past, misremembered or not. It's always with us *right now.* Mari Ruti (2017) stresses this potential marked by zero through revisiting Lacan's version of the death drive (as repetition, excess negativity, symbolic mortification) and his metaphor of the potter who makes a vase "just like the mythical creator, ex nihilo, starting with a hole" (p. 121). "Lacan," she writes, "stresses that emptiness and creativity—the zero of the death drive and the will to begin again; the void of the vase and the fashioning of the vase that comes to enclose it—arise simultaneously" (p. 126). This kind of conjuring generates the gap or impossibility by its own work in responding to the formal lack or impossibility as such (of which *il n'y a pas de rapport sexuel is the most recognizable formulation).* And this contingent presence now resists the nostalgic reduction to a lost object that can be found again. Instead,

[17] See Kelly, K. (2011). *What Technology Wants.* Penguin.

the zero means possibility, potential, as Ruti makes clear. This argument about lack and the zero is largely positive. Writing of Lacan's metaphor of the empty cavity of a vase, Ruti offers: "The zero of the death drive and the hole of the vase are far from being inert spaces of lack. Rather, they give rise to the desire to play with lack; they…generate the impulse to work with negativity" (p. 125).

The possibility opened by this understanding of a fundamental lack (instead of stories of loss) may perhaps upset the iterative future of collecting, of product revision, of the music archive, in favor of the potential for something new:

> Does the future not remain inherently open ended? If so, the subject who turns toward the future by necessity remains alive to the utter unpredictability of existence. This is not a matter of denying death—or even the death drive—but merely of holding on to the possibility that between the present moment and the moment of death we are capable of meeting the world in ways that are worthy of our passion. (p. 119)

This inclination toward the future would seem to be in keeping with Lyotard's (1984) description of the postmodern as "that which denies itself the solace of good forms, the consensus of a taste which would make it possible to share collectively the nostalgia for the unattainable" (p. 81). But here, well into the twenty-first Century, some of us are already nostalgic about the postmodern condition, a theory-time before the vast present of archive soup and product iteration vacated the future. Of course—as an abdication of responsibility Ruti described in the previous chapter—that postmodern past can be a fantasy, too. But if we keep its historicity in mind, perhaps it's maybe also not so bad as nostalgias go. A reflective kind of nostalgic longing, according to Boym (2011), "does not follow a single plot but explores ways of inhabiting many places at once and imagining different time zones.… At best, it can present an ethical and creative challenge, not merely a pretext for midnight melancholies." We can use ethical and creative challenges.

References

Aristotle. (1991). *On rhetoric: A theory of civic discourse*. Oxford University Press.

Armstrong, R. (2013, March 7). Where did the future go? Warrenellis.Com. warrenellis.com.

Benjamin, W. (1969). *Illuminations: Essays and reflections* (H. Arendt, Ed.; H. Zohn, Trans.). Schocken books.

Boym, S. (2002). *The future of nostalgia*. Basic Books.

Boym, S. (2011). Nostalgia. *Atlas of Transformation.*. http://monumenttotransformation.org/atlas-of-transformation/html/n/nostalgia/nostalgia-svetlana-boym.html

Bridle, J. (2011, March 21). Starpunk. *Booktwo.*. http://booktwo.org/notebook/starpunk/.

Ellis, W. (2009). *Shivering Sands* (First Edition ed.). International Electrophonic Unit.

Ellis, W., & Rodriguez, I. (2008a). *Doktor sleepless volume 1: Engines of desire*. Avatar Press.

Ellis, W., & Rodriguez, I. (2008b). "You will never own a jetpack: Warren Ellis' Doktor sleepless. In *Doktor sleepless #7: Marg Bar Amrika* (p. backmatter). Avatar press.

Fink, B. (1996). *The Lacanian subject*. Princeton University Press.

Gibson, W. (2003). *Burning chrome* (Reprint ed.). Harper Voyager.

Goldsmith, K. (2012). *April 26*. Poetry Foundation; Poetry Foundation. https://www.poetryfoundation.org/harriet-books/2012/04/the-new-aesthetic-and-the-new-writing

Gunkel, D. J. (2000). *Hacking Cyberspace. JAC, 20*(4), 797–823.

Holt, N. (2009, January 6). *Love Me, Love My Doll* [Video recording]. https://www.youtube.com/watch?v=f59N37xH0Ng

Irigaray, L. (1985). *This sex which is not one*. Cornell University Press.

Jeffries, A. (2012, November 1). Warren Ellis on futurism, the new aesthetic, and why social media isn't killing our children. The Verge. https://www.theverge.com/2012/11/1/3569208/warren-ellis-futurism-new-aesthetic-social-media

Kornbluh, A. (2024). *Immediacy: Or*. Verso.

Lacan, J. (1999). *Encore: On feminine sexuality, the limits of love and knowledge* (J.-a. Miller & B. Fink, Eds.; 1st edition). W. W. Norton & Company.

Laslocky, M. (2005). *October 11.* Just like a woman. https://www.salon.com/2005/10/11/real_dolls/
Loveless, N. (2019). *How to make art at the end of the world: A manifesto for research-creation.* Duke University Press.
Lyotard, J.-F. (1984). The postmodern condition: A report on knowledge (G. Bennington & B. Massumi, Trans.; 1st edition). University Of Minnesota Press.
Metzger, D. (1995). *The lost cause of rhetoric: The relation of rhetoric and geometry in Aristotle and Lacan.* SIU Press.
Miller, J.-A. (2008). Extimity—The symptom 9. https://www.lacan.com/symptom/extimity.html.
Murphy, J. (2018, October 22). *Why are robots and corpses so creepy?* Welcome to the Uncanny Valley. https://www.mdlinx.com/article/why-are-robots-and-corpses-so-creepy-welcome-to-the-uncanny-valley/lfc-2852
Rao, V. (2012). *April 19.* Hacking the Non-Disposable Planet. https://www.ribbonfarm.com/2012/04/18/hacking-the-non-disposable-planet/
Ruberg, B. (2022). *Sex dolls at sea: Imagined histories of sexual technologies.* MIT Press.
Ruti, M. (2017). *The ethics of opting out: Queer theory's defiant subjects.* Columbia University Press.
Silver, V. (2008, January 2). *My fake baby [video recording].* True North Productions.
Soler, C. (2006). *What Lacan said about women: A psychoanalytic study.* (J. Holland, Trans.). Other Press.
Sterling, B. (2010, February 10). Atemporality for the Creative Artist. Wired. https://www.wired.com/2010/02/atemporality-for-the-creative-artist/
Tomšič, S. (2015). *The capitalist unconscious: Marx and Lacan.* Verso Books.
Vardhan, H. (2024, April 16). "AI girlfriends will build $1 billion industry," *US CEO Predicts Amid Growing Digital Romance.* Mashable India. https://in.mashable.com/science/73360/ai-girlfriends-will-build-1-billion-industry-us-ceo-predicts-amid-growing-digital-romance
Žižek, S. (1997). *The plague of fantasies.* Verso.
Žižek, S., & Critchley, S. (2007). *How to read Lacan (1st edition).* Norton & Company.

7
Failure

Almost half a century ago, Lyotard (1984) claimed, "We have paid a high enough price for the nostalgia of the whole and the one, for the reconciliation of the concept and the sensible, of the transparent and the communicable experience" (p. 81–82). While the ways in which we're charged may have changed, we still keep paying that price.

Fantasies of the whole, the complete, the available and satisfying object of desire keep the engine of capitalism racing while we feel like we're stuck. As Mark Fisher (2009) describes, the capitalist-realist situation "is more like a pervasive atmosphere, conditioning not only the production of culture but also the regulation of work and education, and acting as a kind of invisible barrier constraining thought and action" (p.16). Horizons have been shortened, choices constrained such that the future is evacuated and the present is an enduring hectic stasis.

Trapped in the totalizing frantic oscillations of sameness, it's no wonder that we sometimes look to the past for a difference, for half-remembered feelings of not being caught, of possible futures that were still possible. These futures haunt us. But so often, nostalgia for different options than we have now—or futures we've lost—turns to mythic totalities of race or nationality or whatever and in the coupling of the

T. Richardson, *Nostalgia, Fantasy, and the Futures of Masculinity*, The Palgrave Lacan Series, https://doi.org/10.1007/978-3-032-23921-1_7

"apprehension of loss with a rediscovery of identity and especially of a national community and a unique and pure homeland—we often part ways and put an end to mutual understanding" (Boym, 2011). Fantasies of the complete and whole (past, present, or future) encourage conservative ideologies of gender (and race and nationality) that foment fear, anger, and violence.[1]

I'm not sure how we stop paying the price of such nostalgia, at least at the level of policy and politics. Totalizing gestures toward stasis like digital music archives (or artificial intelligence, or The Internet), repetitive oscillations of capitalist discourse, fantasies of loss and reclamation, et cetera, all seem unavoidable and reinforce feelings of helplessness and loss. But I think exploiting the breaks we can find in the whole—those available means of persuasion—is a strategy worth pursuing. Hacking as "particular practices and movements that only become manifest through specific performances" suggests a direction (Gunkel, 2000, p. 799). If banking on the whole and the one can be resisted, it can maybe be responsibly resisted only contingently and locally.

In relation to consumer capitalism, I suppose that one response could be buying local, or from websites offering hand-made artifacts instead of mass-produced objects: farm to table; Etsy over Amazon. Supporting the individual entrepreneur over the corporation seems right. But wouldn't this be another market appropriation of individuality, much like punk from the shopping mall? And in this stage of late capitalism, where the marketing of the self seems both necessary and inevitable, entrepreneurship may be another *personalizing* of the desire on which the discourse of capital relies.[2]

Extending Foucault's entrepreneurship of the self, Byung-Chul Han (2015) posits personal assumption of capitalist discourse this way:

---

[1] These fantasies also promote conspiracy theories, since everything must always already have a place in the whole. For more on conspiracies in other terms, see Rice, J. (2020). *Awful archives: Conspiracy theory, rhetoric, and acts of evidence*. Ohio State University Press.

[2] In the sixth grade, our son was forced to take a course in "entrepreneurship" in which they mostly watched old episodes of the television show *Shark Tank* (2009), wherein hopeful entrepreneurs pitch their ideas to a panel of celebrity investors.

> The late-modern achievement-subject is subject to no one. In fact, it is no longer a subject in the etymological sense (subject to, sujet à). It positivizes itself; indeed, it liberates itself into a project. However, the change from subject to project does not make power or violence disappear. Auto-compulsion, which presents itself as freedom, takes the place of allo-compulsion. (p. 46)

Pressure from outside (*allo*) is translated to pressure to achieve (*auto*) that feels like it comes from within, an extrinsic force tamed by the fantasy called freedom that's so important to the fundamental fantasy of a complete and autonomous self. For Lacan, the bar (lack, impossibility) is constitutive of the subject and guarantees that the subject is not an object and is always contingent and provisional. The *positivizing* of the subject described above as its *liberation into a project* is thus the eliding of the bar and a subsumption of the subject into the "free" market. This liberation into a project is the project of neoliberalism. So, the translation of the subject discussed in other terms in the second chapter via the capitalist discourse here takes on its full dimensions. Not only is my desire now caught in the circulations of capital, I feel wholly dedicated to a pursuit that is both foreign and homely.

Capitalism depends on the fantasy of a true (positive) self that just needs to be actualized. This is the positivizing of the subject into a project. "Personal responsibility" and "freedom" depend on this fantasy, often linked to a nostalgic recollection of when these were self-evident (when men were real men and pulled themselves up by their own bootstraps; documentation of this is often old movies, themselves totalizing fantasies belying a foundational impotence). And today's social media influencers—entrepreneurs of the self *par excellence*—offer *authentic* living via idyllic images of moving off the grid and driving in customized vans away from the pressures of the market. As Tiziana Terranova (2022) writes, "Instead of the hacker, the 'influencer' has become the new heroic figure" (p. 10). By promoting an authentic life (authentic by what measure?), these influencers extract value from self-care for the social media marketplace.[3] The result is that, As Anna

[3] In some ways, this is about deploying fantasy in its conservative function. Benjamin (1969) argues: "The growing proletarianization of modern man and the increasing formation of masses

Kornbluh (2024) explains, "In constant pursuit of reputational capital to shore up their contractor profiles, individual laborers are rendered 'auto-entrepreneurs', self-employees who charismatically radiate their intrinsic value" (p. 34). Maintaining the appearance of intrinsic value becomes an all-encompassing pursuit, as everything is content such that "when presentation is personalization, when all content is self, when experience trumps idea, any dimensionality, ambivalence, or ambiguity disappears. As a result, tension and contradiction are excluded; only opposition remains" (p. 60). Vaccines are bad and bananas are good. Simplifying choices should mean making life easier. And we could all do with some easier. But "Control only works if you are complicit with it," so while choosing to buy small and local may *feel* better, that *feeling* is the marketing point (Fisher, 2009, p. 22).

Even more in the spirit of the contingent and local, I sometimes spend weekend mornings trawling local estate sales, often searching for the kinds of vintage stereo equipment mentioned in the first chapter. While this kind of buying has the benefit of keeping stuff out of landfills and maybe financially helps families who've experienced a recent loss, the fact that *in every case* I don't need these things, along with the combination of the mortuistic and the bargain, can make me feel icky and sad.

Feeling icky and sad is pretty common these days. So is feeling angry, confused, and just tired. As Mark Fisher (2009) maintains: "To a degree unprecedented in any other social system, capitalism both feeds on and reproduces the moods of populations" (p. 35). The amplification of whatever feelings I have is also now market driven. Outrage is a cultural obsession in part because I know I'm being short-sheeted and also because television and the internet all tell me it's the maid's fault. Or, often, that Generation Whatever doesn't know how to make

are two aspects of the same process. Fascism attempts to organize the newly created proletarian masses without affecting the property structure which the masses strive to eliminate. Fascism sees its salvation in giving these masses not their right, but instead a chance to express themselves. The masses have a right to change property relations; Fascism seeks to give them an expression while preserving property. The logical result of Fascism is the introduction of aesthetics into political life. The violation of the masses, whom Fascism, with its Fuhrer cult, forces to their knees, has its counterpart in the violation of an apparatus which is pressed into the production of ritual values." (p. 241) beds. Byung-Chul Han (2017) argues that "consumer capitalism operates through the selling and consumption of meanings and emotions" (p. 46), not particular objects, and it's not difficult to see how my own buying is so often regulated by grocery-store-shopping my feelings or by staging retreats from *the real world* in order to recharge. Maybe I need a van? Or maybe a cruise?

Or maybe I don't have to go anywhere, as Mari Ruti (2017) suggests:

> Consider the common practice of using online pornography to take a "break" from work, to recharge one's ability to tackle the next task, or to endure the dullness of the day. From this perspective, pornography is an efficient tool of biopolitical conditioning, perhaps even the epitome of neoliberal efficiency: you take your break, there is no emotional mess—the mess being limited to the physical surfaces of your immediate surroundings—and then you go back to work, back to the performance principle. The libido, in this scenario, is not repressed but instrumentalized in the service of increased productivity.[4] (p. 62)

While pornography is a funnier example, any so-called "break" from work is now just as masturbatory, as instrumentalizing even my little time away succeeds in extracting value in the form of increased productivity. I never need to leave my office. We see this in exercise facilities and food courts on corporate campuses, of course, and especially in the lunch-break internet shopping I enjoy while eating at my desk. The invisible hand job of the market.[5]

Maybe *buying* is never the best means of resisting that old restorative nostalgia. If global, national, and even state politics feel hopeless,

---

4 Alenka Zupančič (2017) discusses *Anti-Sexus*, a fictional brochure by Marxist writer Andrei Platonov describing a device that is designed "to isolate, extirpate what is sexual about enjoyment, from all other pleasures and relations in which it appears—to distillate, as it were, the pure essence of sex (and then administer it in just the right dosages)" (p. 28). The promise is that such a device would free users from the pressure of sexuality to allow for both more "meaningful" relations and increased productivity (meaningful relationships and productivity be roughly the same, I guess).

5 Alenka Zupančič (2017) borrows the phrase from Aaron Schuster, and adds "The invisible hand of the market, supposedly looking after general welfare and justice, is always also, and already, the invisible handjob of the market, putting most of the wealth decidedly out of common reach" (p. 32). Here, I think, we also find the libidinal investment of Crypto Bros and the support capital provides for that aggressive version of failed masculinity.

local politics is often less ideological and more practical. Potholes and such. Pushing for—or even just voting for—policies that promote anti-capitalist values like shared public space and the de-privileging of private (and corporate) ownership may allow room for the kind of exploration and discovery that could open the potential that's already here. Shannon Mattern (2021) makes this policy point when arguing for public libraries:

> As an institution that has long been committed to patron privacy, and one that is increasingly embracing principles of digital justice, libraries can—and must—position themselves as "spaces of exception" to exploitative digital urbanism. Frequently romanticized as "oases" amid urban clamor and commercialization, libraries are perhaps instead more like "special epistemological zones" (kind of like less devious, less capitalist "special economic zones") that resolutely embody unsmart knowledge politics and uphold the ideals of inclusion, equity, and justice above efficiency, convenience, profit, and the tangle of compromised values undergirding capitalism in its various permutations: racial, platform, surveillance capitalism, and so forth. (p. 81)

These "special epistemological zones" could offer not just temporary respite from the pressures of capitalism that have colonized even our private time, but would also encapsulate an exception (an extrinsic space) within the neoliberal body itself. The traditional "liberal" values related to the public good on which public facilities were founded—and that Reagan-and-Thatcher-era neoliberalism began to smother—here may resurface as new potentials. But these already-existing spaces allow for the unpredictable—and are potentially useful—only if the totalizing force of value extraction is thwarted. If the future is to remain open, then we have to also resist defining success via the kind of "growth" that is really the cycling of capitalism. These sites need to fail the market. And even if nothing major, earth-changing comes from a local manifestation of the potential that is a library, here in the Texas heat, having someplace cool indoors that doesn't require me to buy something is good-enough reason to keep them safe.

Such spaces belong to neighborhoods. Specificity of place, along with responsibility to the folks who use the space, are paramount. Too often, the future that's styled for us is a featureless, corporate one promising that I can do my job anywhere and feel pretty much the same. The experience of sameness is never indigenous and expands stasis to geography as well as time. Mark Fisher (2014, 2022) talks about the colonization of local specificities with a spatial ennui:

> Public space has been consumed and replaced by something like the third place exemplified by franchise coffee bars. These spaces are uncanny only in their power to replicate sameness, and the monotony of the Starbucks environment is both reassuring and oddly disorientating; inside the pod, it's possible to literally forget what city you are in. What I have called nomadalgia is the sense of unease that these anonymous environments, more or less the same the world over, provoke; the travel sickness produced by moving through spaces that could be anywhere. (p. 137)

What Shannon Mattern (2021) calls "vital local, embodied, situational forms of intelligence" (p. 17) that make up a specific, historical city are replaced with anonymous anyplaces that for some may make travel pointless because they feel like they never left. Furthering the promise of "friction-free capitalism," this kind of beige colonization finds a counterpart in technologies that promise the end of commuting by making my home my workplace (Gates, 1995, p. 181). I don't need a jet pack if I don't need to go anywhere. If I'm comfortable, I never have to stop, especially if I can get Authentic Mexican Food delivered to my doorstep. And since I'm always connected, I can freely work from *any* home. I should feel grateful.

I'm not grateful, and not just because my best years are behind me. Frustration is the low-level hum behind my daily (in)activities. If, as argued variously in the previous chapters, ideology banks on an established system of desires to which I'm asked (or forced) to subscribe to give life order, then the kind of subject I've been reaching for throughout pushes back. Instead of belief in the system—the fundamental fantasy of the whole and the one—this subject is defined by the *failure* of interpolation. Once I give up allegiance to an authentic subculture, piece of cake, masculinity, or robot doll, living with and in the failure-to-consolidate that fantasy tries to cover is the best option open. Instead of a summing maxim that soothes or distracts, I'm left with, to borrow from Lacan (1999), "Nothing but the effects of those instances of saying" (p. 46). By denying the positivizing belief in an essential truth—the myth of the primal father, original greatness, whatever—what's left is mostly relational, contingent, present as effects, and thereby actionable.

But I don't know what those actions should be. Here, I can but echo Keller Easterling (2021):

> This would be the customary moment to announce a new right answer in manifesto form. But against everything culture holds dear, on the other side of that trapdoor, nothing is new, nothing is right, nothing is free, and there are no dramatic manifestos, ur-enemies, or universals. That conforming move, though perhaps labeled "radical," would be sadly conservative. (p. 7)

Nothing is new, nothing is right, nothing is free, and there are no dramatic manifestos, ur-enemies, or universals. Still, doing something feels necessary. Throwing up my hands and acquiescing would be tantamount to assuming the fundamentalist (and the fetishist) perspective, "I know it is not really true, but I believe in it" (Žižek, 2022, p. 212). Still, what should I do?

A lot of this book has been devoted to discussions of sexuality—masculine fantasy, belief versus masquerade, sex dolls and robots—because, following Alenka Zupančič (2017), "when—in the human realm—we come across something and have absolutely no clue what it is, we can be pretty certain that it 'has to do with sex.' … there is sex only in something that does not work" (p. 23). And "Sex is real because it marks an irreducible limit (contradiction) of the signifying order" (p. 46). Sex is the name that, following Freud, Lacan gives to the impossibility that this book has been drawing out. That is, the failure of the whole and the one and the lie of the fundamental fantasy, especially as this fantasy is demonstrated through nostalgia and/of masculinity (masculinity and capital both premised upon a belief that covers failure). The failure of the whole can be seen through the little gaps that mark it, and it's in the gaps—the failures—that action is possible.

After asking what sexuality is, Zupančič answers bluntly and provocatively: "Far from chaining humanity to its animal or natural heritage, sexuality is the problematic territory of being that seems to throw us out of joint, disorient us, and make us indulge in things characteristic of human society (politics, art, science, love, religion ...)" (p. 35). Politics, art, science, love, religion, etc., are active responses to what has been described variously in this book as impasse, impossibility, split, gap, and failure. And these activities are failures that—at their best—generate more opportunities to fail.[6]

I mean fail in a useful way. At the heart of these kinds of activities is a cause that eludes proper naming[7] and instead drives curiosity about relations and possibility. Here, I follow Jack Halberstam (2011) in asserting that

> failure allows us to escape the punishing norms that discipline behavior and manage human development with the goal of delivering us from unruly childhoods to orderly and predictable adulthoods. Failure preserves some of the wondrous anarchy of childhood and disturbs the supposedly clean boundaries between adults and children, winners and losers. (p. 3)

Failure avoids the orderly and predictable, and avoiding takes work. Easterling (2021) calls this kind of work *medium design*, suggesting that, "Rather than prescribing solutions, like buildings, master plans, or algorithms, medium design works with protocols of interplay—not things, but parameters for how things interact with each other" (p. 10). Easterling continues: "Transposing from a nominative to an active register, the intent of designing interplay is not to fix positions but to initiate interactivity" (p. 11). At a very local, personal-historical level, the exchange of cassette tapes described in the first chapter demonstrates the kinds of

---

[6] Brian Eno (1996) argues that "The importance of symbolic behaviours like art and religion and sexual fantasy is that they allow us to experiment symbolically with new and even prohibited positions on the axial matrix—experiments that may be inconvenient, dangerous and divisive in 'real life'" (p. 302).

[7] Keller Easter begins her book by asserting "Culture is very good at pointing to things and calling their name, but not so good at describing the chemistry between things or the repertoires they enact" (p. vii)

interactivity a medium can open up. In the gaps between, in the tensions produced by contingent relationships and the affordances offered by new alignments, something can happen. Maybe.

In *How to Make Art at the End of the World* (2019), Natalie Loveless argues for robust research-creation activity to allow room for academic curiosity beyond the disciplining of disciplines:

> It is an erotic, driven, invested practice. And, as such, it fails to fit into those models that see interdisciplinarity as a way to streamline and multiply research productivities. It is too disruptive for that. Research-creation follows desire, and builds spaces and contexts that allow the time and space to experiment in unpredictable directions. (p. 70)

The aim of her project is to make room for a kind of academic inquiry that reaches beyond disciplinary boundaries as it needs to, following curiosity rather than

> the ways that the disciplined university, with its merit boards and granting agencies structured to assess faculty outputs on the basis of contribution not to 'new knowledge' in general but to new knowledge within a discipline, often renders those who would work practicetheoretically…both illegible and, in the most hostile of assessments, suspect (p. 28).

The mechanisms that support research and the production of "new knowledge" also ensure the reproduction of the disciplines. In so doing, universities and their apparatuses—much like the high school cliques discussed in third chapter—enforce the boundaries on which their cohesion-through-exclusion relies. Just as markets constrain choices to a few models to infinitely delay satisfaction (while at the same time generate public desires that we take as personal deficits), product-driven research very often produces an expected product for which a space on the shelf is waiting. This means, of course, that for a job, for tenure, for promotion, for health insurance and basic needs, any work had better always already fit that space. With no room—and no time on the clock—for curiosity and experimentation with the attendant possibilities of failure, all work had better be conservative work. Nobody gets fired for buying IBM.

Discipline or curiosity. Rigor or failure.

Discipline and rigor are often nostalgic. As Halberstam (2011) writes, these kinds of terms "signal a form of training and learning that confirms what is already known according to approved methods of knowing, but they do not allow for visionary insights or flights of fancy" (p. 6). In my own field, so many of the policies inflicted on our students—seminar papers, comprehensive exams, the prescriptive dissertation—are defended through fond recollections of the well-meaning hazing we had to get through ourselves, but now tied to the more recent mania for networked Learning Management Systems, data-driven discovery, artificial-intelligence proficiency, and standardized assessment introduced by the neoliberal-ized university. The result is a new onanism described by Byung-Chul Han (2017) as "digital networking and communication have massively amplified the compulsion to conform" and "numbers and data are not just being absolutized—they are becoming sexualized and fetishized" (p. 88, 65).[8] The systematic belief that the whole may be captured through numbers (dollars, data points, whatever) means that any failure is always a personal failure to live up to the models. *Model* is another name for fantasy.

But the point that needs to be insisted on is that, nostalgically or otherwise, this situation isn't unavoidable. As Wendy Hui Kyong Chun (2015) reminds us, "if something stays in place, it is not because things are unchanging and unchangeable, but rather because they are continually implemented and enforced" (p. 158). Implementation and enforcement are what ideology is all about.

Thus, the *personal* failure to apprehend the object of desire is valuable because it marks the failure of the person as a unified (ideological) subject. If there is no authentic self to recapture, if we give up the notion of successful consolidation—the whole and the one that Lyotard denigrates—then we're left with a not-whole and boundaries we can trespass.[9]

---

[8] And returning us to the discussion of the pornographic in the previous chapter, Han (2017) writes: "This amounts to nothing other than libidinal energy flowing into today's 'Quantified Self'. On the whole, dataism is displaying libidinous—indeed, pornographic—traits" (p. 59).

[9] That is, feminine sexuation. These are the two sides of sexuation and, as Calum Neill (2020) reminds, "The crisis in masculinity consists in the fact that it is a position predicated on an impossible assumption of self-identity" (p. 16)

This means taking up the object cause of desire (*objet petit a*) not as something that has been lost that must be recovered in a fantasy of completeness, but as a goal I will always fail to reach, as an asymptote of desire, as a direction to explore and not a home to return to. There is no original piece of chocolate cake that must be recaptured, but an opening of possibilities regarding what a piece of chocolate cake can be. This reorientation of the object,

> articulates the drive in the mode of aim rather than attainment.... The objet petit a gives us orientations and lures, rather than prescriptive models of practice. It is the thing that grabs our curiosity, but that we can't quite comprehend from where we are situated, and so off we go in pursuit .... (Loveless, 2019, p. 85)

I love this notion of pursuit. And it could be a breathless pursuit, a life-long "erotic, driven, invested practice" (p. 70). Embracing the lack as an aim then "enables us to overcome the stupid self-contended life-rhythm, in order to become 'passionately attached' to some Cause—be it love, art, knowledge or politics—for which we are ready to risk everything" (Žižek, 2000, p. 108). I want to be passionate about a pursuit, not jog on a treadmill in the workplace gym.

The kind of work Loveless and Žižek (and Easterling and Zupančič) are talking about is ultimately creative. Exploring the newly-opened possibilities that eliding the unified subject allows means forging new, sometimes even previously-prohibited connections that in turn make radical change—even the end of capitalism—conceivable. Jacques Lacan (1988) understood the creative prospect of traversing the fantasy as far back as the mid-1950s:

> That the subject should come to recognise and to name his desire, that is the efficacious action of analysis. But it isn't a question of recognising something which would be entirely given, ready to be coopted. In naming it, the subject creates, brings forth, a new presence in the world. (p. 228–29)

This new object isn't something that I receive from others, but one of my own choosing. It depends on neither a first piece of cake nor a last cigarette, but is instead contingent and active now as a new aim and new possibility. And it's this new object Lovelace (2019) claims "we are in the grip of when we find ourselves pushing our projects into disciplinary and formal directions that we don't yet know how to justify" (p. 84).

I am not at all suggesting that we each need to undergo psychoanalysis to fix the world. Or, alternatively, that we all become artists. But I think, along with Easterling (2021), that I need to be doing everything I can to remain open to unforeseen potentials, "not the ossified consensus that is often the goal of power and the end of politics, but the destabilizing of aesthetic signals as they bounce through culture" (p. 18). Success is too often measured by consensus. That's why trophies are made in advance. Against this ossified consensus, then, I must continually reaffirm the impossible and unknown and make sure that there is always room for failure.

The special epistemological zone that Mattern describes above could be a space that allows for experimentation and failure, that doesn't rely on the discipling nostalgia of the past or future, but constantly engages with the past and the future as generative failures. After all, the past has failed to maintain itself in the present and the future has failed to appear. What we're after is action that "is not predictive, but it does nourish an imagination that manipulates potentials as well as events. And to consider these latent potentials in space is to begin to work around the modern mind" (Easterling, 2021, p. 28). That "work around" is the work worth doing.

To repurpose Lacan's (1990) pun, we are all *homme-sick* (p. 5). Conspiracy theories, climate change denial, etc., are head-in-the-sand responses to the real breaks in the cycles of production that capitalism depends on and that some people enjoy. The insistence on STEM in schools is really often an insistence on participation in the cycles, and increasingly, denying Science and Math (which can also point to the breaking) pushes the positivism of Technology and Engineering. Everything is a nail and we just need better hammers.

Can we change our relationships with the loops of nostalgia and markets that make up the modern mind and fail, as Halberstam (2011) argues, "as a refusal of mastery, a critique of the intuitive connections within capitalism between success and profit" (p. 11)? Maybe a classroom could be the kind of epistemological space for this working-around? Maybe.

Both of our kids have gone through public primary and secondary education and have rarely been allowed to be curious, to explore (except early on when they were encouraged to look for a vocation to dedicate themselves to). Instead, most often, they were taught to the test and credentialing, with attendant graphs and plot points alongside traditional report cards. This data mattered for tracking them as students, sure, but even more for their teachers and schools in terms of jobs and funding from the state. It's hard for the powers to extract value from curiosity because curiosity depends on failure and has no timeframe.

Colleges and universities are not in any way immune to the quantification of what is increasingly becoming solely vocational education. Measuring worth in growth and fiscal value means relegating anything that costs to failure.

It could be useful (but not profitable) for our classrooms (especially our Humanities classrooms) to offer, in Easterling's (2021) words

> extra-political and aesthetic capacities in spaces of interplay—the latency, indeterminacy, entanglement, heavy information, failure, temperament, and discrepancy that the modern mind abhors. It is an endeavor that may not be for everyone. Instead of seeking solutions alone, you can address dilemmas with responses that do not always work. Multiplying problems can be helpful. Messiness is smarter than newness. Obligations are more empowering than freedom. (p. 18)

Failure, temperament, discrepancy, and the rest mean assessments that evaluate (and re-evaluate) process and not product, investment and not return.[10] For the instructor and the student, personal responsibility—that old saw that marks an impossible failure of ideology—has to be reimagined as Haraway's (2016) call to response-ability: "learning to be truly present, not as a vanishing pivot between awful or edenic pasts

[10] A modest example: using an adapted version of the portfolio-based assessment called The Learning Record, an older returning student in a recent course was able to "get credit" for learning how to use the presentation software that every other student in that course had grown up with. Under a results-only system, this learning would have been unaccounted-for labor.

and apocalyptic or salvific futures, but as mortal critters entwined in myriad unfinished configurations of places, times, matters, meanings" (p.1). And this other kind of rigor would need to move beyond the classroom, into workplaces, living rooms, online, everywhere since, as Easterling (2021) maintains, the goal isn't "designing a thing, but rather the means to engage, unwind, infect, hijack, or rewire an arrangement over time" (p. 19). That time may be longer than a semester. It could life-long. Maybe.

Anna Kornbluh (2024) frames the problem and a possible response thusly:

> Though a genuine psychic emergency and a genuine stuckness underlie the imprisonment in the imaginary and hence the enjoyment of immediacy as style, the genuine response to such a situation must be more rather than less mediation—more arts and ideas, more ambiguity and adumbration. No matter how trendy or expedient, opting to drown in the extremity of bad affects without the punctuating relation to an other, to propagate immersiveness against contradiction, and to circulate ever more egoic image can do little but hinder working through. New constructions, new signifiers, new bases for connection, new orders of sociality can emerge only from mediation, not immediacy. (p. 63)

Mediation means denying the supposedly authentic self—in terms of blame or merit—for the mess of working through and toward a sociality that can effect change. When Jodi Dean (2025) calls for a national investment universal basic services ("education, transportation, and health care") and their public support ("libraries, museums, and the arts"), this means attention to medium, to movement, to work without a final cause (p. 143). This is a privileging of care. Maintenance. Collective action begins with focusing on the medium, the action. My suspicion is that this work has to take place locally, exploiting affordances we already have to show new potentials. In municipal buildings, in classrooms, but also in backyard workspaces, in kitchens, and on vacations. This is a kind of serious play.[11]

Working

In any case, I've stopped asking my students about the music of the past, at least directly. Since I already knew what I wanted them to say, that line of questioning felt as if it put them on the spot. My recent appeal has been to ask them to share sounds—musical or otherwise—that mean something to them. From there, we might then ask how and why they mean anything? What were the material conditions. If it's a song, what medium first gave it to you, where and when, etc.? If it's another kind of sound…? How would you make those conditions now in order to reproduce the sound? How would this version be different? The same kinds of questions can be asked about writing, painting, whatever. I don't know what their answers will be, and that feels both exciting and a little dangerous. The idea is to get at local and contingent ways to draw attention to the gaps and then exploit these gaps.

As academics, we are experts in not knowing. We teach how not to know and how to want to know more.

So much of this book has been about stasis and cycles, about being trapped and believing I'm not. Due to the coincidence of late capitalism and my late middle age, giving in to the restorative kind of nostalgia that promises return to a mythic peace and happiness is so tempting, as is being angry at everyone who seems to stand in the way and for whom realizing that fantasy would bad. Product, political, news, and work cycles feel inescapable. In response, I remind myself what Mari Ruti (2017) maintains, that even in the grip of these cycles,

[11] It's cliché, but I remember the first time I saw Star Trek cosplayers—including an original series red-shirt—at a Renaissance festival. Their presence drew attention to the rampant anachronisms and inaccuracies already present in the squashing-together of centuries and emphasized other ways the past and future can be narratized. No one was mad. But the point is that we don't even have to time travel. Just shift among now-possible nows.

> there is room for a degree of "rebirth" in the sense that each new cycle of the repetition compulsion repeats slightly differently—draws new elements, new debris of life, into the groove of the compulsion—so that even when the repetition is largely predictable, it is always also somewhat unpredictable; to the extent that something new is added to the repetition compulsion with every new enactment, one can still speak of a "fresh start" of sorts. (p. 125–26)

This *something new*—the gaps that appear in the whole—mean that the potential for change is nascent in everything that seems unsurmountable. That's the hope, at least. And the debris of life in the locked record-groove of compulsion, or the loss of fantasized fidelity marked by the tape-hiss of desire as failure, opens the possibility of a future that hasn't already been counted. Debris insists on the present by implicating the past as past. By amplifying whatever breaks up the fantasy of the whole and by assuming responsibility for that noise, we can maybe set up the conditions for a future that will have been better.

References

Benjamin, W. (1969). *Illuminations: Essays and reflections* (H. Arendt, Ed.; H. Zohn, Trans.). Schocken books.

Boym, S. (2011). Nostalgia. *Atlas of Transformation.*. http://monumenttotransformation.org/atlas-of-transformation/html/n/nostalgia/nostalgia-svetlana-boym.html

Chun, W. H. K. (2015). Crisis, crisis, crisis; or, the temporality of networks. In R. Grusin (Ed.), *The nonhuman turn* (pp. 139–166). Univ Of Minnesota Press.

Dean, J. (2025). *Capital's grave: Neofeudalism and the new class struggle*. Verso.

Easterling, K. (2021). *Medium design: Knowing how to work on the world*. Verso.

Eno, B. (1996). *A year with swollen appendices*. Faber and Faber.

Fisher, M. (2009). *Capitalist realism: Is there no alternative?* Zero Books.

Fisher, M. (2022). *Ghosts of my life: Writings on depression, Hauntology and lost futures* (2nd ed.). Zero Books.

Gates, B. (1995). *The road ahead* (First ed.). Viking Press.

Gunkel, D. J. (2000). Hacking Cyberspace. *JAC, 20*(4), 797–823.

Halberstam, J. (2011). *The queer art of failure* (Illustrated ed.). Duke University Press.
Han, B.-C. (2015). *The burnout society (1st edition).* Stanford University Press.
Han, B.-C. (2017). *Psychopolitics: Neoliberalism and new Technologies of Power* (E. Butler, Trans.). Verso.
Haraway, D. J. (2016). *Staying with the trouble: Making kin in the Chthulucene* (First ed.). Duke University Press.
Kornbluh, A. (2024). Immediacy: Or, The Style of Too Late Capitalism. Verso.
Lacan, J. (1988). *The seminar of Jacques Lacan, book II: The ego in Freud's theory and in the technique of psychoanalysis, 1954-1955.* Norton & Company.
Lacan, J. (1990). *Television.* Norton & Company.
Lacan, J. (1999). *Encore: On feminine sexuality, the limits of love and knowledge* (J.-a. Miller & B. Fink, Eds.). W. W. Norton & Company.
Loveless, N. (2019). *How to make art at the end of the world: A manifesto for research-creation.* Duke University Press.
Lyotard, J.-F. (1984). The postmodern condition: A report on knowledge (G. Bennington & B. Massumi, Trans.). University Of Minnesota Press.
Mattern, S. (2021). *A City is not a computer: Other urban intelligences.* Princeton University Press.
Neill, C. (2020). Masculinity in crisis: Myth, fantasy and the promise of the raw. *Psychoanalysis, Culture & Society, 25*(1), 4–17.
Ruti, M. (2017). *The ethics of opting out: Queer theory's defiant subjects.* Columbia University Press.
Terranova, T. (2022). *After the internet: Digital networks between capital and the common.* MIT Press.
Žižek, S. (2000). *The ticklish subject: The absent Centre of Political Ontology.* Verso.
Žižek, S. (2022). *Surplus-enjoyment: A guide for the non-perplexed*. Bloomsbury Academic.
Zupančič, A. (2017). *What IS sex?* The MIT Press.

Index

T. Richardson, *Nostalgia, Fantasy, and the Futures of Masculinity*, The Palgrave Lacan Series, https://doi.org/10.1007/978-3-032-23921-1

FSC
www.fsc.org
MIX
Papier | Fördert
gute Waldnutzung
FSC® C083411

Kolibri 360 GmbH
Ferdinand-Jühlke-Straße 7
99095 Erfurt, Deutschland
produktsicherheit@kolibri360.de